Cruising Crew

Cruising Crew

How to be welcome on board

Malcolm McKeag

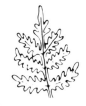

Fernhurst Books

First published in 1991 by Fernhurst Books, 33 Grand Parade,
Brighton, East Sussex

Printed and bound in Great Britain

British Library Cataloguing in Publication Data
McKeag, Malcolm
    Cruising Crew: how to be welcome on board
    1. Sailing
    I. Title
    797.124

ISBN 0-906754-63-1

Acknowledgements
The author and publishers would like to thank the Westerley Sea
School and Rosie Kempner for providing yachts for photography,
Motor Boat & Yachting for providing a camera boat, Tim Bartlett for
driving it, Kathy Braund, Susan McKeag and Christine Graves for
crewing on camera, and John Mellor for all his help and advice.

Photographs
All photographs by Julia Claxton, with the exception of the following:
Andrew Bray: page 14 (top).
Tim Davison: page 6.
John Driscoll: page 19 (right).
Tim Hore: page 24 (top), 26, 41 (top), 43 (bottom), 68–69 (bottom), 72,
75 (bottom), 76, 77, 78 (left), 80.
Kos: cover
Motor Boat & Yachting magazine: page 33, 44, 93.
John Woodward: page 18, 19, 20, 21, 41 (bottom), 45, 49, 90 (left), 95
(top).

Edited and designed by John Woodward
Composition by Central Southern Typesetters, Eastbourne
Artwork by PanTek, Maidstone
Printed by Ebenezer Baylis & Son, Worcester

Contents

Introduction   7

1   Welcome on board   8

2   Looking after yourself   16

3   Meet the hardware   22

4   Ropework   30

5   Getting going   33

6   Sailing along   40

7   Tacking and gybing   52

8   Lowering sails   60

9   Sail changing and reefing   65

10   Spinnakers   72

11   Arriving   81

12   Emergencies   90

Glossary   96

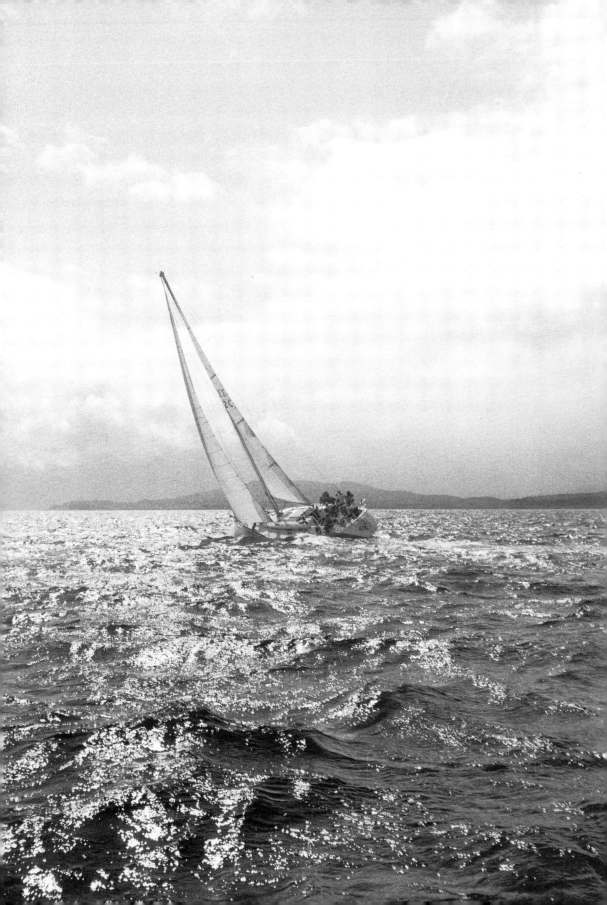

Introduction

There can be no such thing as 'the complete' guide to being a member of the crew of a cruising yacht. This book makes no such claim, and has no such ambition. Any competent cruising crew will tell you there is more to working a yacht than can be put in one book.

So this book confines itself to one main aim: overcoming the strangeness of stepping aboard a cruising yacht for the first time. Avoiding that uneasy feeling of apprehension as she puts to sea with those around you speaking a language from another planet; the embarrassment of having to ask, in what is always too public a moment, how the toilet works; the sense of helplessness, not to say rising panic, that affects you the first time she trails her rail to a sudden squall.

Several aspects of cruising that might merit a book of their own are hardly touched on here, for they simply do not concern a first-time crew. Other topics, some might say, have been laboured beyond measure – but that is because what seems obvious to an expert is far from obvious to a beginner. Certainly, there are things mentioned in these pages that neither the author nor the publisher has ever seen in any other book. That was a principal reason for writing the book in the first place.

Although there is often a wrong way to do things aboard a yacht, there is seldom only one 'right' way. Some skippers like a thing done one way, others like it done another way. You may use a method shown here and find that your own skipper likes things managed differently; that does not mean that either this book or your skipper is wrong. Hopefully, no one will disagree too violently with a method shown or an opinion passed here.

In particular, ways of doing things have to be adapted to the gear you find on the yacht you join. Yachts vary so much in detail that it is impossible to be wholly precise in a general book. A large part of the art of seamanship is making the best use of the tools and gear at your disposal.

Throughout these pages it is assumed that the reader knows virtually nothing about sailing theory and practice, but is keen to learn. So the text explains the basic concepts before dealing with crewing tasks in all the detail necessary to perform them properly, using any technical terms that may be appropriate. Most of these terms are explained in the opening chapters, but if you are in any doubt refer to the glossary.

If by the end of the book you feel more at home aboard a sailing yacht, it will have succeeded in its principal aim. If, having read it, you return from your first sail itching to get out there again, it will have done rather more. And if, as a result of reading it and learning something from it, you are asked back again, it will have been worth every penny of its price and every minute of the time it took to write.

1 Welcome on board

Cruising yachts are as diverse in design as houses. The vast majority have common features but the details differ, depending largely on the size of the yacht. All cruising yacht design is an exercise in squeezing a quart into a pint pot, and the more pint-sized the boat, the more squeezing has to be done.

Starting below deck and right forward we find what used to be called the fo'c'sle and is now – certainly in modern designs – described as the forecabin. Forty years ago (and a well-kept cruising yacht designed forty years ago is not considered old; yachts age much less quickly than, say, cars) the fo'c'sle on a small yacht was somewhere to stow the sails, the anchor chain and similar paraphernalia. Any berths would probably be pipe cots (like camp beds, each with a canvas mattress strung across a four-sided tubular frame). Today there are strong marketing pressures to fill every available space with beds, and a more modern yacht will probably have a vee-shaped platform across the fo'c'sle area of the boat (good children's berth, or for close friends who do not mind entangling their feet) or two proper upholstered berths.

The main constraint on layout in this part of the yacht is the need to deal with the mast and the loads it imposes. If the mast is deck-stepped (the base or heel of the mast rests on the cabin top) there will be a main bulkhead across the boat underneath, literally to prevent the roof caving in. If the mast is keel-stepped it comes right through the boat at this point and the accommodation has to be worked around it.

In the classic layout, the toilet compartment (which on ships and boats is called the heads) would be here, with perhaps a full-length hanging locker (so called because it provides hanging space for clothes) opposite.

Aft of the main bulkhead lies the saloon, usually the main living space. Layouts vary, but usually there are built-in settees which have stowage space under them, with more small lockers against the yacht's sides. In all but the largest yachts the main saloon settees double as regular berths, so at some stage of the on-board day the sitting room has to convert to someone's bedroom.

Adjacent to the saloon are the galley and the navigation area. This latter may be little more than a fold-down table with some adjacent book

⇨ Plan of a typical 30-foot yacht. The settees in the saloon can be converted into berths at night.

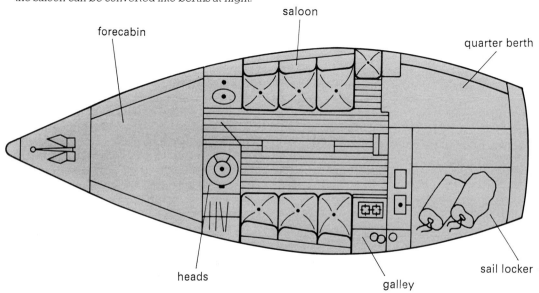

forecabin

saloon

quarter berth

heads

galley

sail locker

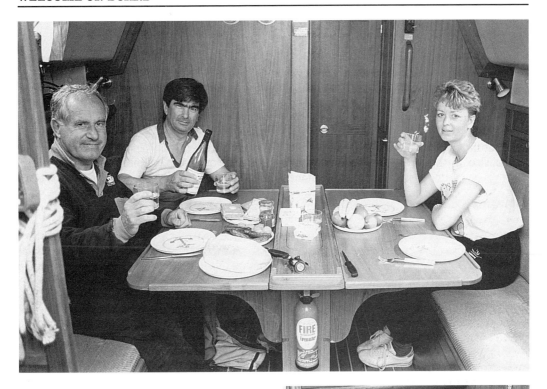

⌂ *The saloon by day. Welcome aboard!*
◊ *A saloon settee used as a berth, and (below) the chart table and navigation area.*

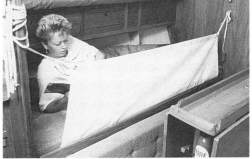

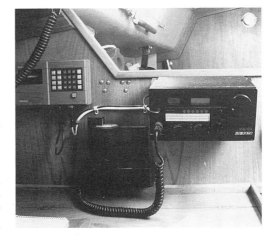

stowage, but on a larger boat it could be a fully-fitted work station. In most yachts the navigation space comprises a built-in desk (the chart table) and seat, the chart table having a hinged top and a half-height bulkhead to isolate it from the main living space.

The opening from the cabin to the cockpit is called the companionway, and the steps up into the cockpit are the companionway steps. Under them will probably be the engine, operated by remote control from the cockpit.

There may be one or two berths slotted in here, under the cockpit. They are known as the quarterberths, not because they offer short measure but because this part of the vessel, between amidships (mid-way between bow and stern) and the stern is known as the quarters.

Since the mid-1980s designers have taken to rearranging the conventional layout just described. The fashion is to design yachts with more beam (width) than before, giving more room down below, and to make the boat higher out of the water. This allows more headroom below, especially aft. It is now common to place the heads aft of the companionway on one side, and create a second cabin (third if you count the saloon as a separate cabin) under the cockpit area. Headroom to one side is provided by cleverly designed 'hollow' cockpit coamings and the double bed is placed under the sole (floor) of the cockpit. There is of course no headroom over the bed, since you are not expected to want to stand up there.

STOWAGE

Space is always at a premium. There will be stowage spaces under most of the berths, with specific stowage spaces for many special items from the spare anchor and liferaft to torches and tools. Much of the smooth working of even an informally-run cruising yacht depends on routine, and neat, assigned stowages are part of that routine; you should always know precisely where to put your hand on a torch in the darkness, for example – and so should everyone else – so putting things back in their allotted stowage is very important. The very word stowage means more than mere storage; it implies that something is not just 'put away', but put away and at the same time readily available when needed.

It is vital that there are marked stowages for the emergency equipment. Hopefully you will never need it, but it should be pointed out and its use explained to each new crew member before his or her first sail. If such a demonstration is not offered to you when you arrive on

---

THE MARINE TOILET

Yachts have no mains water supply and no main drainage, so the marine toilet (known for historical reasons as the head or heads) works on a quite different principle to the one in your home. It is effectively a specialised, oddly-shaped pump, or to be precise two pumps: one for pumping the flushing water in, and one for pumping the waste out. The waste may go straight out into the sea via a closable valve in the hull, or it may go into a sealed holding tank in the bilge to be pumped out at a sewage pumping station.

Most sea-going yachts are equipped with the type that pumps directly into the sea. The method of operation varies from make to make, but the basic problem is the same: getting water in and out when you want to, and stopping it coming in at all other times. There will be two valves – known as seacocks – one for the inlet pipe and one for the discharge. Before using the toilet you must check that both are open by finding the relevant pipes and tracing each from the bowl to its seacock. The valve is open when the lever is turned to line up with the pipe, or if it has a wheel, when the wheel is unscrewed to leave a lot of screw-thread showing.

Having checked the valves, examine the pumps. The simplest types have a back-and-forth lever pump for the inlet and a much larger barrel pump (T-handle, up and down) for the discharge. If there is any resistance on either, then the seacock is closed; further determined pumping will only blow the pipe off the valve, inside the boat. Messy.

Some types have a single lever which operates both pumps. Another design has a single lever and a rubber seal under the seat and lid: working the lever with the lid open empties the bowl, but working it with the lid closed creates a vacuum which draws in the flushing water.

Common courtesy, not to say common sense, demands that the owner or a regular crew member should show you how to work the head before you need it.

Remember that it is really just a large pump, relying on some quite small internal moving parts. It can easily become blocked, and unblocking it is a most unpleasant task. Apart from toilet paper, NEVER PUT ANYTHING DOWN THE TOILET THAT YOU HAVE NOT EATEN FIRST. Fag ends, sanitary towels and even tampons must be disposed of elsewhere.

board, ask for one. You have every right to feel uneasy about going to sea with anyone who offers the slightest rebuke to such a request.

Other specific stowage areas will be found around the galley, for everything from food to the dust-pan and brush. If there is no actual fridge with a conventional opening door there may well be an ice-box: a well-insulated, deep cavern with a drain at the bottom where perishables may be kept cool when stowed with bags of ice.

Shore-going clothes are usually kept in the hanging locker, the yachting equivalent of a wardrobe. Inevitably this will be much smaller than any wardrobe, and although it will have enough depth to take a jacket on a hanger, it will not take a ball-gown.

ELECTRICS

Yachts do not have mains electricity, unless there is a supply laid on at the mooring, and this means that household appliances do not work aboard yachts. Most yachts have either 12-volt or 24-volt electrical systems, used principally to power navigational equipment, navigation lights and cabin lights – in that order of priority. The power comes from a battery or batteries (usually stowed securely under the navigator's seat) which are charged by the engine – and only when the engine is running. Using electricity when the engine is not running therefore drains the batteries: you will be expected to use it sparingly, switching off anything (such as cabin lights) that you do not actually need.

There is normally a master switch called the battery isolator somewhere in the system; if you switch something on and it does not work, check that the isolator switch is 'on'. Start looking for it (probably a large black or red key-like switch) alongside the engine or on the side of the navigator's seat. To prevent battery drain it is normal to switch off all power at the isolator when leaving the boat, even if you are only going off to the pub for an hour or two.

WATER

Although she may be fitted with taps which produce water on demand, remember that the yacht is not attached to a water main; all fresh water has to be carried in tanks, probably fitted under the main saloon berths or, in a bigger boat, in the bilges. Fresh water, like electricity, must be husbanded and used with discretion. Water pressure is provided by an electric pump, which switches on automatically when the tap is opened.

Habits like leaving the tap running while brushing your teeth will win few friends no matter how bright the resulting smile. And although the heads may incorporate a shower, if you insist on three showers a day you may find that the skipper has removed the fuse from the shower pump.

GAS

Bottled gas is the most commonly-used fuel for cooking, although solid fuel systems and systems using paraffin oil are not unusual. The gas bottle will probably be stowed on deck or in a special locker with its own drain leading directly overboard, the gas being fed to the cooker through a flexible pipe. In addition to the taps on the cooker itself there will be a tap on the top of the bottle and another somewhere in the system, between the bottle and cooker and usually just to hand.

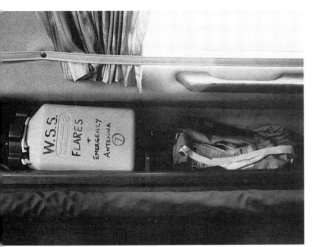

◊ *Stowage for flares and lifejackets at the back of a saloon berth. Be sure you know where all emergency equipment is stowed.*

There is a very real danger of accidentally leaked gas gathering in the bilges and causing an explosion as soon as someone lights a match or even causes a spark by switching on an electrical appliance. To minimise the risk the gas should always be turned off at the main tap – not just at the cooker tap – when the cooker is not being used. Many skippers will also insist that you turn off the gas at the bottle every time as well. Needless to say you should never turn on the gas and leave the tap open while you look for a light. If you are distracted and forget, the consequences could be disastrous.

ON DECK

Moving around the deck, safety is paramount. There is an old sailorman's saying 'one hand for the ship, one hand for yourself'; it holds true today as ever. The deck of a yacht is seldom flat even in harbour – there are curves, corners and bumps everywhere – and at sea it rarely stays still for long. Fortunately the place abounds in handholds, but in making use of them make sure you are grabbing something solid, not something such as a rope attached to a sail, which may suddenly move.

The vast majority of modern cruising boats have a 'fence' around the deck: the guardrails, supported by vertical stanchions. At the bow there is usually a solid steel frame known, for reasons which become obvious the first time you see one, as the pulpit. This provides secure support for anyone working on the foredeck.

The most obvious thing on deck is the mast, supported by the rigging. The side rigging wires are the shrouds, while the rigging wires which come to the centreline (fore-and-aft) are stays. The most important of these is the forestay, which runs from near the top of the mast to the bow. The horizontal spar aft of the mast is the boom.

Most modern cruising yachts are sloops; that is they have two fore-and-aft sails: the mainsail and headsail. The mainsail is set on the boom and hoisted up a track or groove on the mast; the headsail is set on the forestay. The yacht may have several headsails of various sizes and weights of cloth to suit differing wind conditions, but only one will be set at a time.

⇨ A typical sloop with an aft cockpit and tiller steering. All the lines are led to the cockpit, allowing the yacht to be controlled in safety and reasonable comfort.

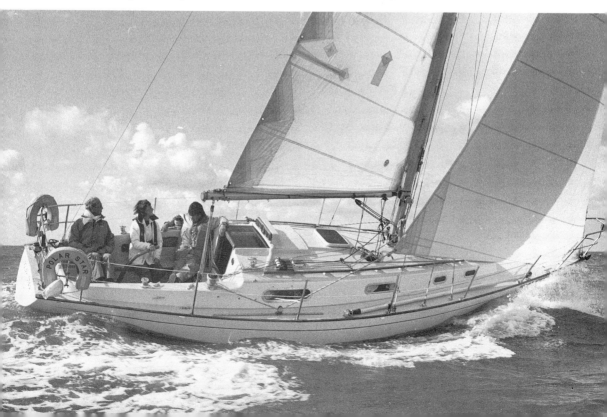

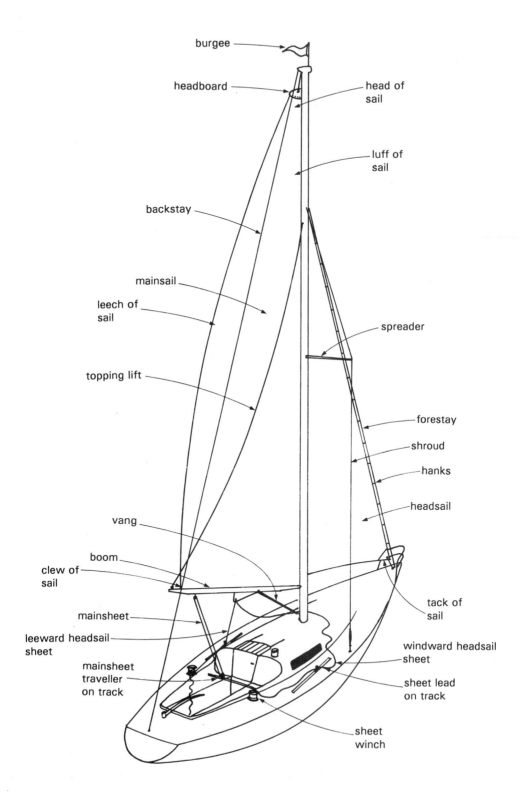

burgee

headboard

head of
sail

luff of
sail

backstay

mainsail

leech of
sail

spreader

topping lift

forestay

shroud

hanks

headsail

vang

boom

clew of
sail

tack of
sail

mainsheet

leeward headsail
sheet

windward headsail
sheet

mainsheet
traveller
on track

sheet lead
on track

sheet
winch

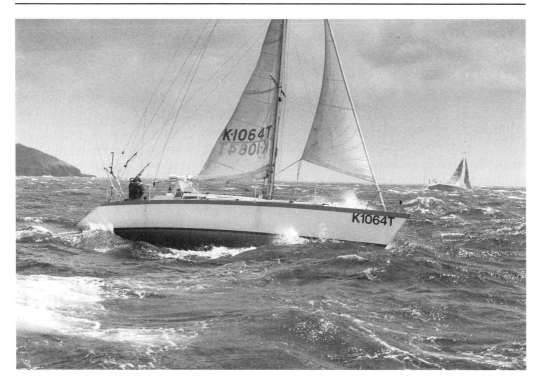

⌐ *A roller-reefing headsail can be part-furled to reduce its size. This yacht also has running backstays.*

⌐ *The author in the cockpit, trimming the mainsail. Note the winch and the row of stoppers in the foreground.*

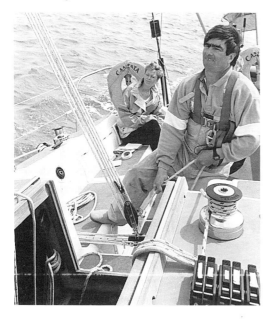

Many yachts now have a roller-reefing headsail. One all-purpose headsail is set permanently on a thin spar which either replaces or fits over the forestay; the spar can be turned by means of a rope-and-drum arrangement at the lower end, enabling the headsail to be rolled and unrolled rather like a roller blind. The amount of sail unrolled is judged to match the wind strength of the moment, largely obviating the need to carry several headsails or to change sails while under way. For sheer convenience the system is a joy to use and can more or less eliminate foredeck work, but there is no doubt that the all-purpose nature of the sail compromises its looks and efficiency. There are few, if any, roller-furling headsails which when part-rolled set as well as a purpose-made sail of the same size.

The ropes or wires which hoist the sails are called the halyards, while the ropes which pull the sail in or let it out are called the sheets. On all but the tiniest yachts the halyards, sheets and most control lines are worked on winches (see Chapter 3). Across the deck near the companion hatch you may find a row of small levers: these are stoppers, which stop-off and secure the lines at their working settings.

The well in which the crew normally work is the cockpit. Here you will find the principal sheet winches and the mainsheet control; this will probably be a block and tackle mounted on a slider set on a transverse track, called the traveller.

You will also find the helm, which is the all-embracing name given to the steering apparatus: it may be a long wooden or metal tiller connected directly to the rudder head, or it may be a wheel, connected to the rudder either by direct linkage (cables or rods) or working through a hydraulic pump.

Right aft, you will find the backstays: probably a permanent backstay mounted on the centreline and corresponding to the forestay, and possibly at either side the running backstays, which have to be set up and released depending on the point of sailing. Rigging which is set up and not normally adjusted is called standing rigging, whereas rigging which has to be adjusted as a matter of course when working the ship is called running rigging, and includes the running backstays, the sheets, halyards and control lines.

LIVING ABOARD

Living aboard a yacht is all about sharing a confined and sometimes cramped space with other people – so consideration of others combined with keeping your own corner in order are the golden rules.

Don't bring so much gear with you that you take up all your own stowage space and overflow into space needed by others; on the other hand you will be a perfect pest if you travel so light that you are always having to borrow sweaters, sun-tan cream or something to read.

Do remember that everything you bring will have to be stowed in small, oddly-shaped lockers, or in your bag which itself will have to be stowed somewhere; don't bring rigid trunks and suitcases which cannot be folded away. Likewise, if you are keen on photography, don't bring your cameras in a hard metal case with sharp corners to knock chips out of glassfibre and woodwork; bring them in a soft padded bag.

Rules about who and what may be in, on or near the chart table vary from skipper to skipper but can sometimes be quite strict, for very good safety reasons. Do avoid leaving your own bits and pieces littering the chart table: for the navigator there are few things more infuriating than coming to work and finding the things he or she needs buried under a litter of other crew-members' sunglasses, cameras, personal stereos, spare reading matter or whatever.

Smoking

The detritus of smoking is often simply not noticed by the smoker but greatly offends the senses of non-smokers. If you are a smoker, do bear in mind the extra constraints imposed by sharing a confined space with non-smokers, and clear up after yourself with scrupulous care. No-smoking-below-deck is a common and reasonable convention.

Alcohol

Cruising is a social and sociable activity, and conviviality plays a major part in its enjoyment, both in the way of a pleasant drink while sailing along and in a trip to the pub in the evenings. Sometimes the whole point of the cruise may be to get to a particular pub. But just remember that alcohol dulls the brain, blunts judgement, plays havoc with physical co-ordination and slows reactions. It is said that of all cruising accidents, those involving late-night return trips in the dinghy from the pub are the most common. It is curious that while we accept that drinking and driving do not mix, we tend to drink like fish when we get on a boat; the potential for accident is no less, and you should be aware of the fact.

2 Looking after yourself

The first daunting prospect to greet a new arrival at any yacht is the problem of getting on board. Even if the boat is alongside a pontoon in a marina climbing aboard requires a technique; if she is lying offshore on a mooring you must add to this technique the ability to walk on water.

In a marina

The guardrails which will hopefully keep you on board once there also act as an effective barrier to getting there in the first place. First, check that things have not been made simple for you by the provision of steps from the pontoon up on to the boat, or a break in the guardrails to permit easy access.

Assuming there are no such conveniences, climb on board at the shrouds, if they are within reach, or at a stanchion. Do not pull yourself up by a wire guardrail. If you are using a stan-

chion, grab it as near the base as you can (the higher you grab it, the more leverage you exert; constant levering can loosen the fastenings, which is why the knowledgable crew comes aboard via the shrouds, which are more firmly anchored).

Place a foot on the toerail and push yourself up; avoid swinging on the stanchion, and put both feet on the toerail *outside* the guardrail. The secret here is to get your centre of gravity over the guardrail as quickly as possible, by leaning the upper part of your body forward.

Once you are securely on the toerail you can think about getting into the boat. Swing one foot over the guardrail, then the other, keeping a secure hold with your hand while doing so. If you have a bag swing it on board first to leave both hands free for getting yourself on board, or get someone else to pass it aboard once you are safe on deck.

⟲ Pass your bag aboard . . .   *Climb up by a stanchion . . .*   *And over the rail.*

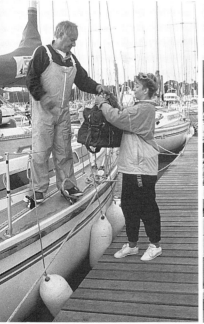
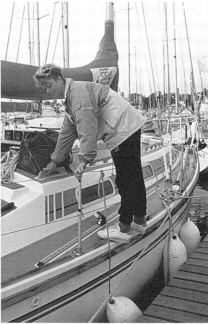
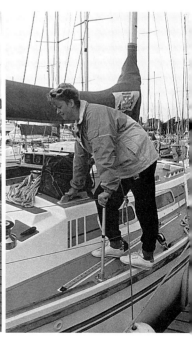

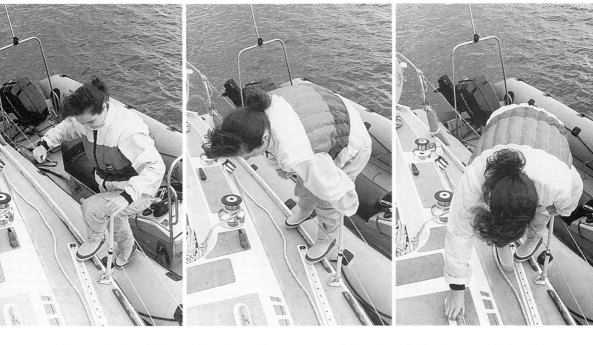

↶ *From a dinghy, climb up by a stanchion . . .*   *Lean forward to get your weight well inboard . . .*   *And swing yourself aboard.*

From a dinghy or launch

The same rules apply, but more so because of two added problems: the boat is that much higher out of the water than the dinghy, and the boat and dinghy will be moving up and down together but out of sequence if there is a swell. Even in flat water, transferring your weight from dinghy to boat will cause the relative levels to shift.

When getting off it is even more important to get both feet on the toerail *outside* the guardrails before trying to get into the dinghy or launch. Resist, at all costs, the temptation to step straight into the dinghy over the guardrail. Sooner rather than later the dinghy you think you are stepping into will move away at the crucial moment and you will be left straddling the guardrail with the top wire between your legs and taking most of your weight. This situation is acutely painful, always undignified and often quite dangerous.

If the height difference is too great to get a foot onto the toerail from the dinghy, launch or pontoon (or vice versa) kneel on the toerail with one knee while effecting the transfer. This is not comfortable, but better by far than falling.

AVOIDING PERSONAL INJURY

You have a responsibility not just to yourself but to your host and your fellow crew members not to get hurt or injured, if only because it will detract from their enjoyment of the cruise if they have to look after you.

Yachts abound with traps for the unwary, and it cannot be stressed too often that thoughtlessness causes more accidents than anything else.

For yourself, never release a rope that is, or may be, under load without making sure you can immediately get your hands free.

Never stand or sit on the down-load side of anything, for fear that whatever is holding it may suddenly let go.

Be careful where you place your feet when working near loose lines and ropes; if they suddenly become loaded, will your foot be inside an ever-tightening loop?

Be especially careful working with wire, for it has a nasty habit of having tiny but razor-sharp 'snags': protruding broken or cut ends of individual strands which can inflict painful wounds.

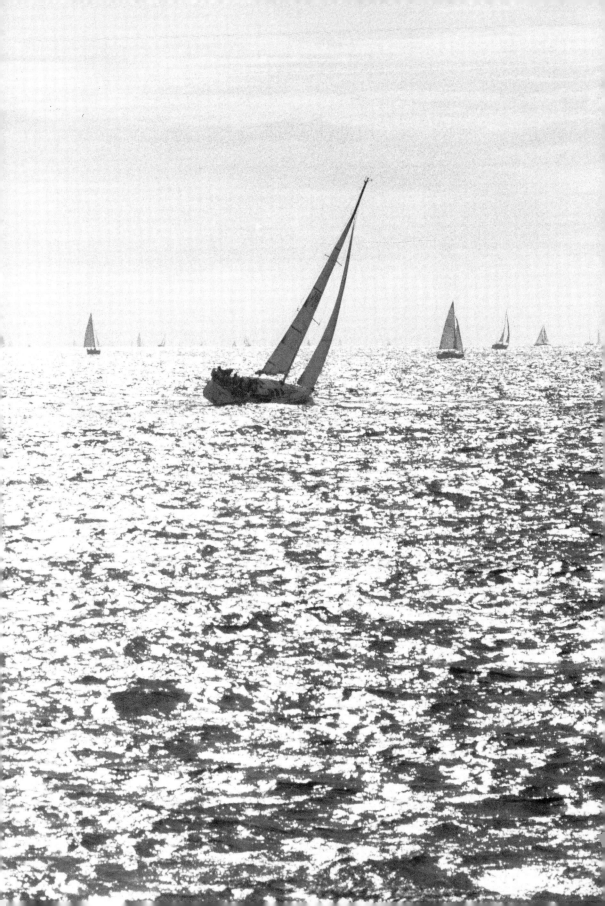

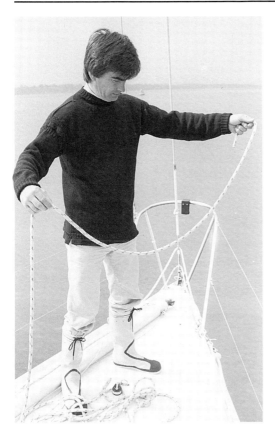

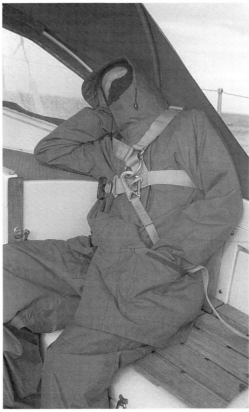

WHAT TO WEAR

Sailing clothing, like ski clothing, combines fashion with function, with the added attraction (for some, at least) of keeping alive some traditional features.

White-topped caps, dark reefer jackets, white trousers and flowing frocks for the ladies are indeed still worn afloat in some circles – but mostly where other people are doing the actual crewing. In the main, comfortable casual clothes are the rule, supplemented by specially-designed heavy weather gear to keep out the wind and water.

In general you should pitch the clothes you wear to the company you will be keeping and to the nature of the outing, much as you would on any social occasion. If you have been asked to join a cruise to rugged parts with plenty of seatime envisaged and the odd trip ashore to some remote pub, the emphasis will be on warm, hard-wearing, comfortable lounging and working clothes. If you have been asked

⌂ You must stay warm, dry and comfortable to enjoy your sailing. A pair of jeans and a sweater will keep you warm, but to stay dry you will need a decent pair of boots, strong waterproof overtrousers (the high bib type are best) and an oilskin jacket with hood.

to join the yacht for a week of day-sailing from one Mediterranean resort to the next, you will want to be able to look presentable in restaurants where the fact that you are an hoary old seadog just arrived on shore from a long sea voyage will cut little ice with the *maitre d'*.

As a rule, though, remember that space is limited, and that even on a fine day temperatures at sea are considerably lower than on land. So take clothes that can be bundled up without creasing or crumpling, and sweaters with a tight weave to keep the wind out. If you stay warm and comfortable you'll have a lot more fun, and be a more useful part of the team.

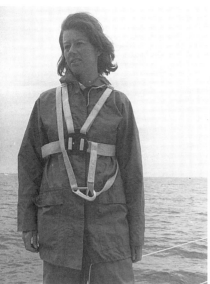 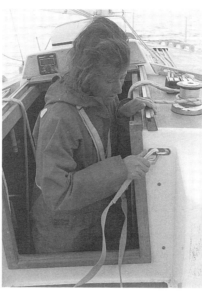 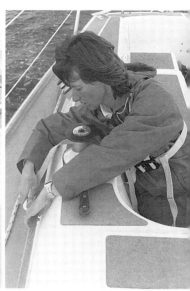

SAFETY HARNESSES

A safety harness is an essential part of your sailing wardrobe. Your skipper will provide it, but it's up to you to wear it and use it.

The harness itself is no trouble – just a bit of webbing with a buckle at the front – so it makes sense to slip it on and keep it on. Make sure it is properly adjusted to fit you – reasonably tight with the buckle over your breastbone – and once you have got it to your liking retain it for the duration of the voyage. Some oilskin jackets have a built-in harness, and if you need to buy a jacket it's a feature worth looking for.

Pass the harness safety line under your left arm and back over your right shoulder, then attach the snap shackle to the line. When you need to use it, you can simply slip the shackle, pass the line back round and clip on.

The boat should be fitted with attachment points in the cockpit for use in rough weather and at night. If you need to go forward along the deck you should clip the line to the jack-stay: a tight wire or webbing strap running the full length of the deck below the cabin windows. The jackstay may run inside or outside the shrouds depending on the yacht's design, but whichever way it runs you must follow the same route as you move forward or the line will foul the shrouds and stop you dead.

Always clip on in rough weather, at night, if

⌒ Always clip on in rough weather and at night. Clip the harness line to the fitting in the cockpit as you come on deck, and transfer it to the jackstay if you have to go forward to work on a sail. And hang on!

you have to work on the open deck out of the comparative safety of the cockpit, and if you are feeling seasick. You are very vulnerable with your head over the lee side of the boat, and while you may not care (in cases of acute seasickness being swept away and drowned may seem like a blessed relief) others will.

Seasickness remedies

Apart from death, the best remedy for seasickness is to get involved in running the ship. Volunteer to steer for a while, watch the horizon and try to ignore the pitch and roll of the boat. If this fails, go below and lie down. Try nibbling a dry biscuit or two.

If you are prone to seasickness, tell the skipper before the trip starts, and he or she will probably suggest a preventative dose of *Stugeron*. It is important to take this in good time, since it will not work if you are already feeling ill.

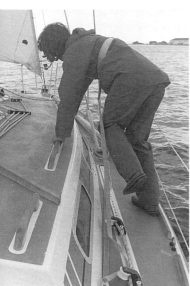
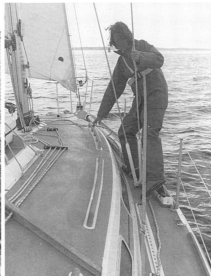
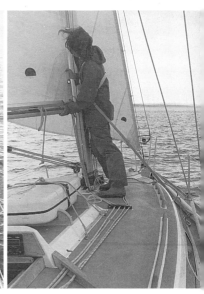

HEAVY WEATHER COOKING

Cooking on board is a tricky procedure at the best of times, but when the sea gets rough it can be dangerous, too. If you are deputed to take your turn in the galley when the boat is leaping around – and it happens to all of us sooner or later – you should take a few essential precautions.

● Use deep cooking pots, and do not even contemplate using the frying pan. If there is a pressure cooker on board use that, with the lid clamped on but unpressurised. Then if it jumps off the stove it will not throw its boiling contents all over you.

● Clamp the pots to the stove, with their handles turned inwards. If the boat has a cheap stove with no clamps, you may be able to improvise with hooked elastic cords – but watch they don't burn.

● Use a minimum of water, and avoid hot oil if at all possible. Both will slop around in a seaway with murderous effect.

● Wear bib-type oilskin trousers to protect yourself, just in case.

● Hang on. The cooker should be fitted with a safety strap to stop you rolling away from it, and a bar to prevent you pitching into it.

● Serve hot drinks or soup in big mugs, half full.

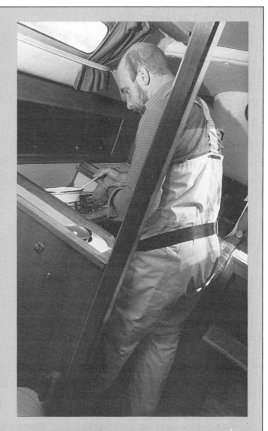

⌂ A galley strap provides hands-free security when the boat is heeling hard.

3 Meet the hardware

Perhaps the most daunting aspect of sailing for any newcomer is coming to terms with the various bits of mechanical equipment found on the average sailing yacht – that, and the fact that almost everything has a peculiar name which rarely appears to have anything to do with the function of the device in question.

WINCHES

The most crucial piece of equipment is the winch, found in some form on virtually every sailing yacht. For the complete newcomer to yachting, one of the sharpest lessons to be learned is the puny strength of man or woman when compared to the weight of the wind in a sail. On a yacht of only 27ft, trying to haul in a drawing sail by simply pulling the rope will achieve little or nothing, while taking it off its cleat or stopper without the mechanical advantage of a winch will result in a nasty fright at the least, and at worst rope-burned palms, crushed fingers and chaos on deck. On a bigger boat the margin for error, and the potential for injury, are correspondingly reduced and in-

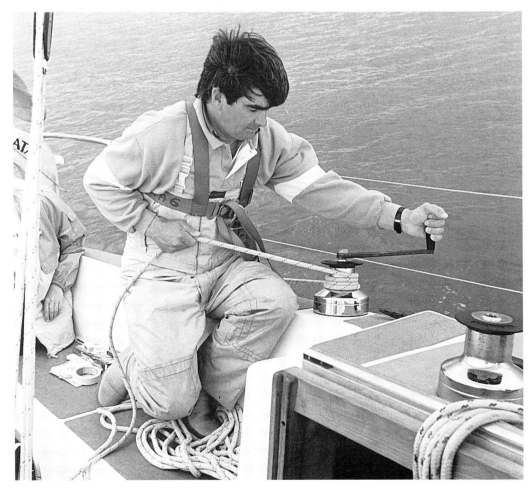

creased. The winch is the basic tool of sail handling; always use one to work a loaded sheet or halyard.

The winch consists of a hollow drum around which a line can be turned (we'll avoid the word wrap – too often it is only too accurate a description). The drum itself is turned by means of a handle, while a ratchet inside the base of the drum allows it to turn one way but not the other. That part of the loaded line which goes into the winch is called the working part, while the length of line which comes off the winch from the turns on the drum is called the tail. A load of great weight can be held on the drum simply by keeping light tension on the tail, provided there are sufficient turns; the load on the working part tightens the turns and the friction of the rope against the drum does the rest. If the load is so great that the rope begin to slip, putting another turn on the winch will often be sufficient to stop it.

Thus the winch allows the crew to hold (snub) a heavy load or, by turning the winch drum with the handle, to haul in a much greater load than even the strongest man could budge. Using the deceptive simplicity of a sheet winch a girl weighing 100lb can easily control a straining sail exerting enough power to haul along a 10 ton yacht.

Mechanical advantage

The mechanical advantage which gives winches their power is provided either by the simple leverage of the handle alone (the longer the handle, the more leverage) or by gearing within the winch. Larger yachts often have winches with two or three speeds; the lower gear is engaged simply by turning the handle the other way, while an even lower gear can be engaged by pressing a button on the side of the winch base before reversing the turning direction again. Combining gearing and a substantial lever arm, the mechanical advantage of a single winch on a 45ft boat might be as much as 65:1.

◊ Winching: take three or four turns around the winch and tension the rope against the barrel while you work the handle with the other hand.
◊ The main winch positions and functions on a medium-sized yacht.

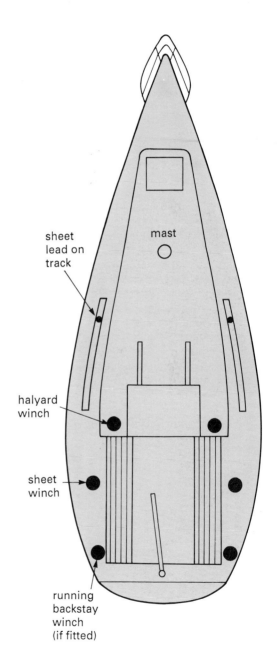

sheet lead on track

mast

halyard winch

sheet winch

running backstay winch (if fitted)

Winch handles

Without a handle a winch can be used only to snub a line; it cannot be used to haul-in. Winch handles are also very expensive, so never leave a handle sitting unattended in the top of a winch; sooner or later a stray line will catch the handle and cause some foul-up. The line could easily flick it over the side, possibly via the face of some innocent bystander.

Older winches – which you may well meet on a cruising yacht built more than 20 years ago – have a slot in the top to take the handle, which is little more than a flat bar. More modern winches have a square or star-shape hole called a key-way which matches the shaped head of the handle.

The simplest handles are solid, but others have a ratchet incorporated in the head, allowing the handle to be moved back half-a-turn to give a more convenient pull. Some handles have a small thumb-lever on top of the head which operates a plate on the underside of the star-key, locking the handle in place in the key-way of the winch head.

Self-tailing winches

Many modern cruisers are fitted with self-tailing winches. These operate exactly like ordinary winches but each has a round, toothed groove on the very top into which the tail of the line is loaded, having first been led over a metal guide bar. As the winch is turned by the handle the toothed groove maintains the tension on the tail and leads it off the winch drum.

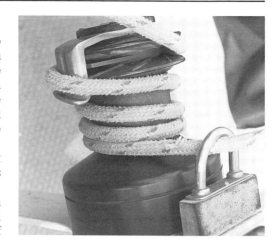

⌂ A self-tailing winch holds the tail taut, allowing you to winch one-handed.

It is important to remember that the actual load is taken by the turns of the line round the barrel of the winch, and not by the grip of the toothed groove on the tail. The tail should simply sit in the groove – indeed if there is any tension on the tail it means that not enough turns have been taken on the drum. Properly, the self-tailer should be loaded with turns all the way from the bottom to the top of the barrel.

Winching

Whether self-tailing or plain, the principles of working a winch are the same; the difference is that with a plain winch you either tail with one hand and wind with the other, or two

⌂ Take a turn round the barrel . . .   *And two more . . .*   *Fit the handle . . .*

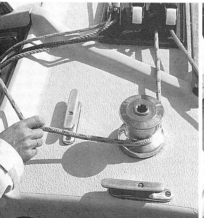
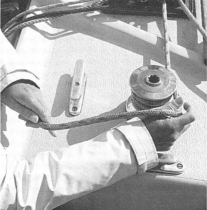
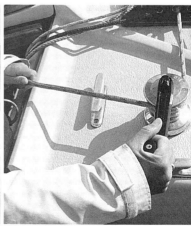

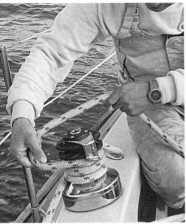 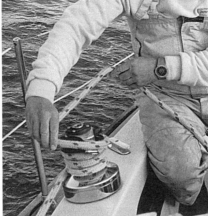 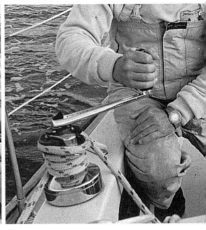

⇧ With a self-tailer, load the winch . . .   *Pass the tail over the guide bar, into the toothed groove . . .*   *And start winching.*

people work the winch: one tailing and the other winding. With a self-tailer, one person can do both – which is why the self-tailer has become so popular. However, a self-tailer is slower to use than a plain winch, especially under light load.

Ensure that the line coming onto the winch is led correctly and does not run foul of anything – the top of the cockpit coaming, for example – and has not been led the wrong side of anything, such as a stanchion base.

The line should rise to the winch at a shallow angle to meet the sloping shoulders at the base of the drum. If the line comes to the winch horizontally, or worse downwards, the line coming onto the winch will ride up over the turns already on the barrel, causing the particular brand of foul-up known as a riding turn.

The winch will turn only one way, usually clockwise; if in any doubt give the winch a quick spin, then put on the turns the same way the winch spins. Just how many turns depends on the job; the heavier the job, the more turns needed. But too many turns can lead to trouble: if the winch barrel is full and you cannot pull the tail off quicker than the line goes on, you may get a snarl-up. Three turns will usually give enough grip for most jobs, and avoids having so much line on the winch that fast-hauling becomes a problem.

Winch in the rope . . .   *Slip the tail round a cleat . . .*   *And jam it.*

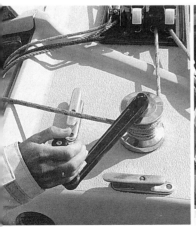 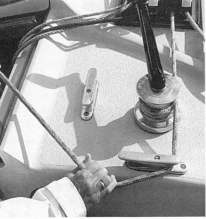 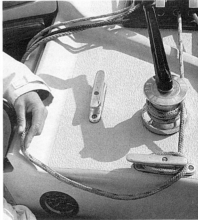

Extra turns

Often – when tacking for example – it pays to have only two turns on to start with, then throw on more turns when the real weight comes onto the winch. This is most easily done with the handle removed. If you can do it before the weight comes on the sheet – Bravo. But you may want to put extra turns on when the load is already on the winch.

The important things to remember are to keep tension on the tail – so the turns already on the drum do not slip – and to ensure your fingers are never on the inside of the extra turn where they could become trapped and crushed between the rope and the drum.

Keep the pull on the tail with your left hand, far enough from the winch to allow the whole new turn to go on without having to move your left hand on the rope. Now put your right hand about two-thirds of the way between your left hand and the winch, and use it to 'push' the line onto the winch, gradually transferring the weight to the line from your left hand to your right.

When your hand is on the opposite side of the winch, twist your wrist slightly to allow the line to go on to the winch without your hand or fingers being on the inside. By now all the load of the tail is being taken by your right hand which is now pulling the remaining line onto the winch. Throughout, the vulnerable fingers of your right hand – the hand nearest the winch – have been on the outside of the line as it goes on to the winch.

⬦ Keep your fingers well clear when taking an extra turn on a winch.

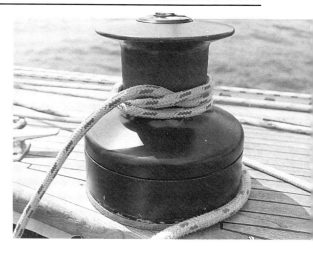

⬦ A riding turn.

Using this method with a self-tailing winch renders the self-tailing device redundant. The alternative is to load the winch completely before you start, but tailing a fully-loaded self-tailer when there is no great load yet come on the line is both dreadfully slow and even harder work than simply hauling off slack line by leaning your weight against it and pulling. The self-tailer comes into its own once the weight is on the halyard or sheet, and the winch is being used for fine trimming.

Riding turns

These occur when line coming on to the winch rides up over the turns already on the drum, either because of a bad lead to the winch or because the tail is not being hauled off the winch fast enough and the line coming onto the winch goes slack. If a riding turn is not spotted quickly, it will jam up the winch completely.

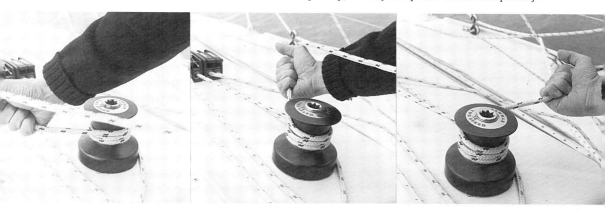

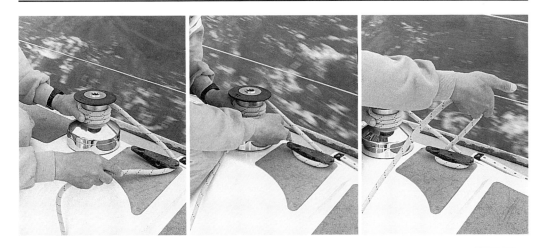

The only way to free riding turns is to take the load off the working part of the line before it comes onto the winch, and remove the turns from the bottom up. If the riding turns occur during a tack (the most usual situation) the only way to free the blocked winch is to rig a temporary sheet to another winch, take the load with that and somehow get sufficient slack into the original sheet to free the turns.

CLEATS AND STOPPERS

Once you have winched in the line, what do you do with it? You need something to hold the tail of the line so it can be left unattended: you need a cleat or a stopper.

Cleats come in a variety of patterns: *staghorn cleats*, round which the line is made up with turns; *jamming cleats*, often with hinged jaws which tighten their grip on the line as the pull on the line increases; and *clam cleats*, originally a trade name but now the generic name for jamming cleats which have no moving parts, where the line is laid into a V-shaped groove which itself has ridged teeth.

Stoppers are basically lever-arm cleats. The line is led through the stopper; when the lever is up the line runs freely, but when the lever is down it presses a toothed cam on to the line to grip it and prevent it running out. Stoppers are often arranged in a bank, each holding its own line, in front of a single winch. The winch is used to work the line which, when set, is stopped-off and unloaded from the winch, freeing it to work another line.

⟳ *To stop a winched line you may only need to take a single turn around a cleat, hauling the tail tight under the forward horn of the fitting.*

When releasing line from jam cleats and stoppers, always do so by first pulling the line on through the cleat or stopper, using the winch if necessary.

⟳ *A line of stoppers securing the halyards and other control lines.*

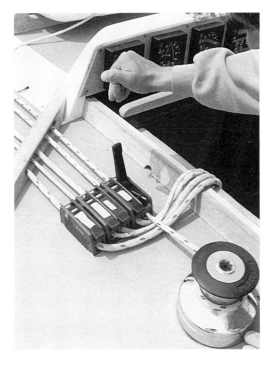

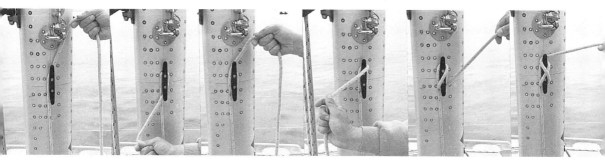

↶ *To make up a line properly on a cleat, lead it round the far horn, put on one complete turn, then criss-cross it and finish with a round turn to jam it.*

BLOCKS

The other principal item used on deck is the block – what landlubbers and ironmongers call a pulley. Blocks come in all shapes, sizes and specialist applications; all basically consist of a smooth wheel (called the sheave) mounted on an axle inside a casing (the sides of which are called the cheeks) over which a line or wire may be led.

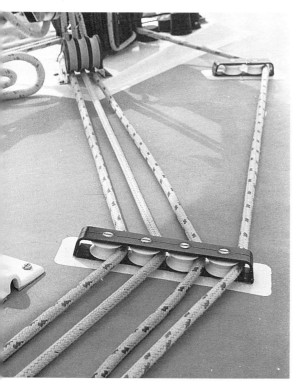

Rigged together, blocks can provide a tackle which can be used to give mechanical advantage (the most obvious example is the mainsheet tackle). Used singly they can alter the run or lead of a line. Some blocks are multi-purpose, while others are designed for just one task; the positions of some blocks are fixed, while others are movable; some are put in place only temporarily to perform an occasional task.

Lead blocks

As their name suggests, lead blocks are used simply to give a fair lead to a line, around a corner or onto a winch. They may be single-sided and bolted permanently in place (called foot-blocks or more simply turning blocks), or they may be ordinary blocks attached to round rings (eye-bolts) on the deck.

The most obvious movable lead blocks are the sheet leads for the headsail sheets, which are usually mounted on a slider which runs on a short solid track bolted to the deck.

Snatch block

A most useful and versatile type of block, this has a hinged cheek so that the line may be put through or removed from the block without having to be led through from one end.

◊ *A bank of turning blocks leading control lines from the foot of the mast.*
↷ *A sheet lead block on its track.*

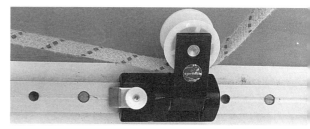

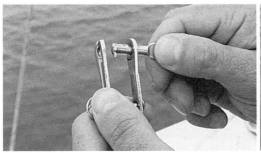 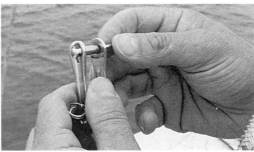

SHACKLES

Shackles are the universal connectors of sailing. Basically, a shackle is a metal U-shaped hoop with a threaded bolt (called the pin) across the open end to act as the closure. It can be used to join more or less anything to anything, provided that each item has a convenient hole through which the shackle can be fitted before being closed with the pin. There are variations of size and shape to suit particular tasks.

The bane of life on board is dropping the pin while trying to hold the two things you wish to connect with the shackle; one answer to this is the so-called safety shackle which has a slight rim round the pin at the threaded end which holds the pin captive even when loose. Another sort of shackle, the key-shackle or quick-release shackle, has a tiny stub (the key) instead of the threads; this fits through a keyway in the shackle, being closed by a half-turn of the pin.

Snap-shackles

These are quick-release connectors. The shackle has an opening hoop, hinged at one end, which can be kept closed by a plunger

⌐ The pin of a quick-release shackle is held captive by the 'key'.

fitting into an eye at the other end of the hoop. Again, they come in a variety of sizes and shapes. Often the plunger has a small loop of line attached to its pulling end, to make working the shackle easier (just as often, it seems, the loop of line goes missing, making the snap-shackle the very devil to open when under load).

OTHER HARDWARE

A handy-billy is a useful device – two blocks with a length of line rove (passed) back and forth between them to give a purchase (mechanical advantage). Each of the blocks has a quick-fitting shackle attached so that the handy-billy can be rapidly fitted wherever it may be needed. It is used for a multitude of short-term tasks about the boat, from acting as a temporary gybe-preventer on the mainboom to hoisting gear out of the dinghy.

⌐ A snap shackle is held shut by a small spring-loaded plunger.

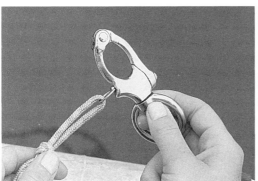 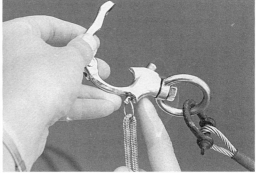

4 Ropework

The first thing you'll notice about any yacht is that there's an awful lot of rope around. and the chances are that the first thing you'll have to do as a new hand is grab one of those lengths of rope, wrap it round or through something and put a knot in it.

In the best-spoken sailing circles knots are either the speed the yacht goes at, or the lumpy things you get in a line which has been left improperly coiled. To a real sailor, a 'knot' is either a bend or a hitch. Generally, a 'bend' is used to join together two lines which will then work together, while a 'hitch' is used to attach a line which is holding something to something else – a post, another line or whatever.

Half hitch

Of itself, this is virtually useless since it comes undone so easily, but it is the basis of many other knots, including the simple bow (as in shoelaces) of which it is the first stage. Everyone who has ever passed one end of a string under the other and pulled has tied a half-hitch. It is mentioned here simply because it is referred to in other knots, below.

Typical use: as a safety hitch, or tying away the free end after forming some other knot such as a clove hitch.

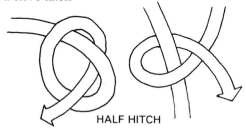

HALF HITCH

Bowline

One of the most versatile of all knots, since all it does is put a soft eye (a loop) in one end of a line. You can tie the loop through something (the clew of a sail, for example, to attach a sheet) or drop it over something (a bollard) or tie it round or over something (such as a post or rail). Its principal disadvantages are that it cannot be untied with the line under load, and

the loop is prone to chafe – which is why it should not be used as a mooring knot. Use a round turn and two half-hitches instead.

Typical use: attaching a sheet to a sail.

BOWLINE

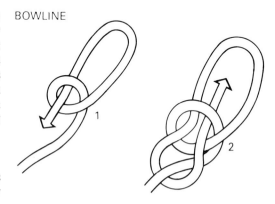

Sheet bend

This is used for joining two ropes together. It is much more secure than the commonly-used reef knot, which tends to collapse under load. If the two ropes are of different thicknesses, form a bight in the thicker rope, pass the thinner one up through the eye, round the back and through. Passing it round the back and through a second time forms the double sheet bend, which is extra-secure.

Typical use: tying a light heaving line to a heavy mooring rope.

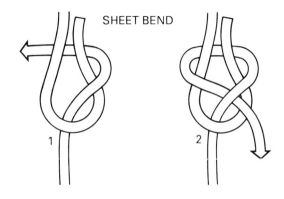

SHEET BEND

Clove hitch

This is for attaching a line to, for example, a horizontal or vertical post. Pass the line over and around the bar, back up over itself and over the bar again, then pass the free end under the second loop. It can also be tied by making two loops and placing one on top of the other, then either dropping them over a bar or post or passing the bar (such as the staff of a burgee) through the two loops. The clove hitch has the disadvantage that it can come loose if it is not under constant load.

Typical use: securing the burgee halyard to the burgee staff (using two clove hitches to prevent the burgee staff toppling).

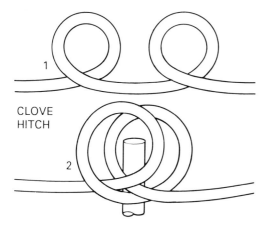

CLOVE HITCH

Rolling hitch

This is much more useful than the clove hitch, since it will resist a sideways pull. The line is tied so that the hitch goes over itself, and the initial double loop 'locks' the line to whatever it is tied to. The third loop simply stops the hitch coming undone.

Typical use: tying a temporary stopper to a line under load (such as perhaps a sheet) while the end of the loaded line is transferred to another winch.

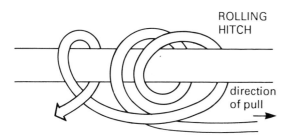

ROLLING HITCH

direction of pull

Round turn and two half hitches

Almost as versatile as the bowline, this is a very simple knot to master. Loop the end of the line over the post or rail, or through the ring, and secure the line to itself with two half-hitches, one behind the other. It has the great advantage that it can be undone with the line under load (although you need to be sure you know what is going to happen once you *do* undo it.)

Typical use: tying a dinghy painter to a mooring ring.

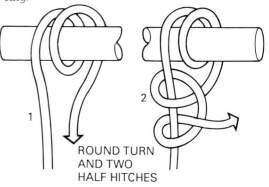

ROUND TURN AND TWO HALF HITCHES

Figure of eight

A nasty knot and one to avoid, yet recommended in many textbooks as the knot to use to form a stopper on the end of a rope to prevent it running through a block. It is shown here so you will know how to undo it and replace it with the much superior stopper knot shown below. Its disadvantage is that if it is used for the purpose intended, it becomes jammed so tight that it becomes nigh-impossible to undo, and may even have to be cut off.

Typical use: demonstrating the superiority of the stopper knot.

FIGURE OF EIGHT

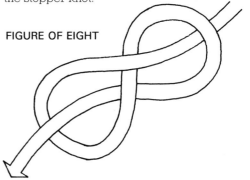

Stopper knot

Form two loops near the end of the line, and pass the end through them. No matter how hard the knot is pulled into the fairlead or block it can later be undone by breaking apart the two loops, which are in fact two half-hitches tied side-by-side.

Typical use: At the end of a halyard, to stop it disappearing up the mast in an unguarded moment.

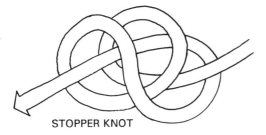

STOPPER KNOT

A neat wrinkle

Here is a neat little wrinkle to make life easier when hoisting the burgee. Usually, the halyard is a light line fed from the base of the mast, through a little block at the masthead, and down again. You attach the burgee on its staff with a clove hitch, then squint upwards as you hoist it aloft. Invariably it goes inside and around itself, and, still squinting upwards, you spend ages twisting and untwisting the two sides of the halyard to get the burgee aloft.

If you untie the knot joining the two ends of the halyard and lead the forward end of the halyard outboard, then forward of the shroud, keeping the other end aft of the shroud, then rejoin the ends, you will never, ever, have to untwist the halyard again. It is amazing the number of people who have never thought of this simple trick.

COILING A ROPE

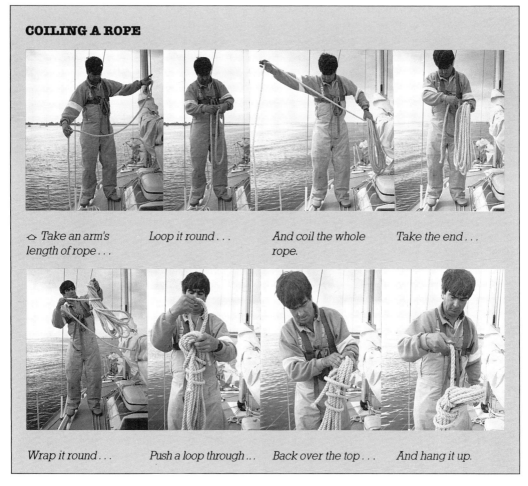

◁ *Take an arm's length of rope...*   *Loop it round...*   *And coil the whole rope.*   *Take the end...*

Wrap it round...   *Push a loop through...*   *Back over the top...*   *And hang it up.*

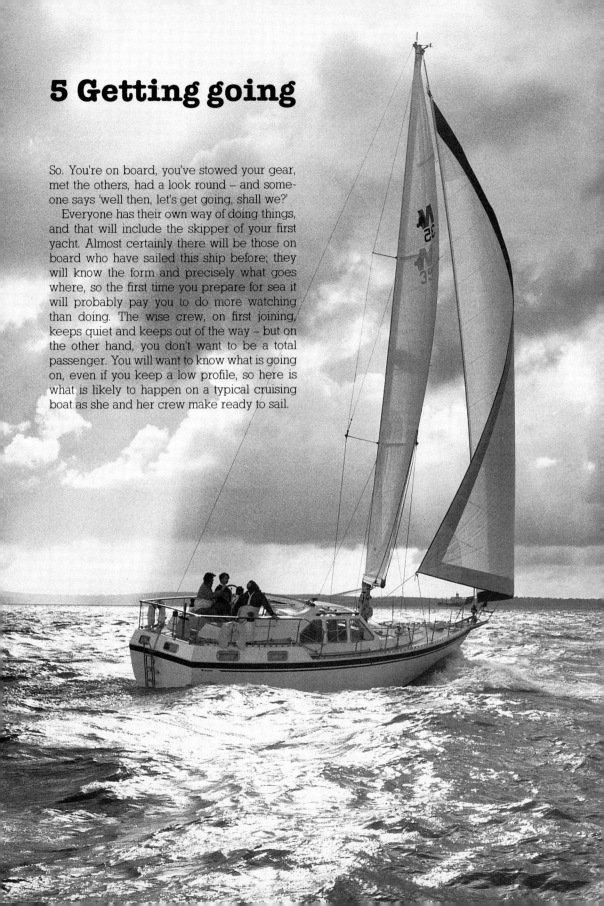

5 Getting going

So. You're on board, you've stowed your gear, met the others, had a look round – and someone says 'well then, let's get going, shall we?'

Everyone has their own way of doing things, and that will include the skipper of your first yacht. Almost certainly there will be those on board who have sailed this ship before; they will know the form and precisely what goes where, so the first time you prepare for sea it will probably pay you to do more watching than doing. The wise crew, on first joining, keeps quiet and keeps out of the way – but on the other hand, you don't want to be a total passenger. You will want to know what is going on, even if you keep a low profile, so here is what is likely to happen on a typical cruising boat as she and her crew make ready to sail.

RUNNING RIGGING

When the boat is parked in her marina berth or on her mooring much of the loose gear and lines will have been stowed below, partly to prevent deterioration and party for security reasons. Sadly, it is a fact of life these days that even in good marinas loose blocks, winch handles and even attractive bits of rope such as jib and spinnaker sheets have a habit of 'walking'.

Winch handles will be unearthed from the cabin and put in their plastic pockets by the winches, and probably on the mast if there are winches there. The sliding roller fairleads for the headsails, plus some snatchblocks used for spinnaker sheets and guys and maybe a handy-billy for use as a foreguy on the boom may have to be put in their proper places. These expensive and eminently removable fittings are often kept in a plastic bucket when the yacht is left unattended, and the first job to be done is bring the bucket on deck and put all the bits and pieces where they will be needed on the voyage.

Unless the boat is fitted with a permanently rigged roller-furling headsail to which the sheets are normally left attached ('bent on', to use the sailorman's term), the jib sheets will have to be rigged. The fool-proof way to do this is to lead them from the cockpit winch, through the turning block that brings the rope onto the winch drum, up the side deck and through the sheet lead block on the slider track, then around the outside of everything to the foredeck. Repeat for the other side, and hitch the two together forward of the mast, ready for attachment to the headsail.

The 'sheets' may be just one length of rope with a small eye-loop, perhaps with a hard eye and a shackle enclosed, at the mid-point where the sheets will be attached to the sail. If this is so you will have to rig them the other way, from the bow. Attach the shackle to the forestay, then lead each 'leg' of the sheet down either side of the boat, reversing the sequence just described.

Check with the skipper that the sheets on this particular boat should be led the 'normal' way; you might get an instruction such as 'inside the main shrouds but outside everything else', or the boat may have several potential sheet leads; the boss will know which one he wants to use today.

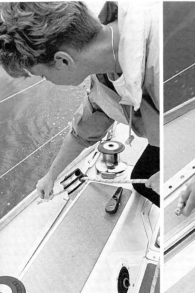
↻ Feed the sheet through the turning block . . .

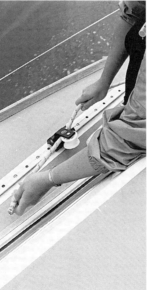
Through the sheet lead block . . .

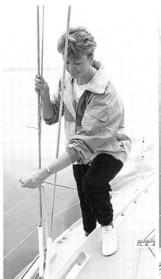
Up the side of the boat . . .

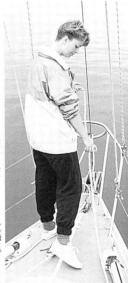
And tie it to the forestay.

MAKING READY THE SAILS

If the sails are not already permanently attached, they must be made ready to hoist.

Mainsail

On most yachts the mainsail is kept permanently bent on to the boom, with a cover to protect it when the boat is not in use. Here's a tip about taking off the mainsail cover: undo the lashing at the mast end last, since that way the cover is less likely to start blowing off when you are half way through the task of removing it. Also, the outboard end of the boom is the least accessible and least secure place for you to work, so you do not really want to be there holding the full weight of the rolled-up cover when you could, with a little more forethought, be enjoying the solid security of working where the boom is rigidly attached to the mast and is easily reached.

Some smaller boats (and many racing boats) take the mainsail right off the boom after every outing. In this case it has to be put on by sliding the foot along the track or groove in the boom, then folding the sail over the boom and securing it with sail ties until the time comes to hoist.

Headsail

Unless the boat has a permanently rigged roller-furling headsail, the headsail will be in its bag below; stowed either in a cockpit locker or, most probably, in the forecabin.

There are two ways in which the sail can be attached to the forestay; either by hooks (known as hanks) which are fitted at intervals to the luff of the sail and which go around the wire forestay, or by fitting the smooth bolt-rope of the sail into the groove of the headfoil – a lightweight metal fairing which fits over the wire forestay.

Many cruiser-racers, and virtually all racing boats, use the headfoil system because aerodynamically it is more efficient and thus improves the sailing performance of the boat. Despite this all sensible cruising yachts not already fitted with a roller-furler headsail use the more old-fashioned hanks. They have the supreme advantage that, once hanked-on, the sail remains attached to the forestay whether up or down. The groove of the headfoil holds the luff of the sail only when the sail is up,

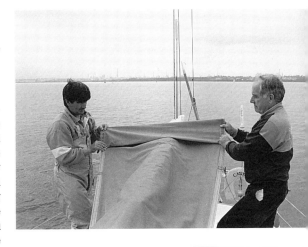

◁ *Roll the mainsail cover from the boom end.*

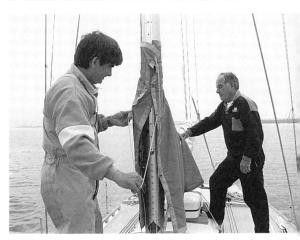

◁ *Unlace it at the mast . . .*
◁ *And roll it back on itself.*

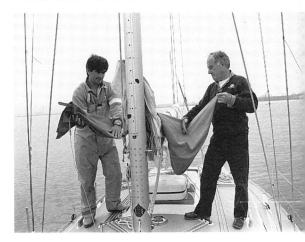

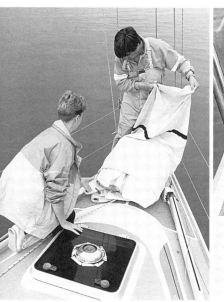
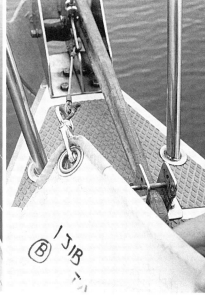
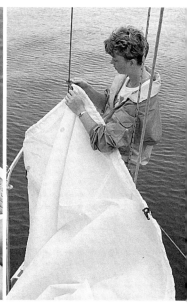

⌂ *Take the headsail forward and out of its bag . . .*

Shackle the tack to the fitting at the foot of the forestay . . .

And start hanking on the sail, starting at the bottom.

leaving it to float around loose at all other times and making handling it on deck a great deal more difficult. Frankly, headfoils on cruising yachts are a real pain in the sterngland.

While we're on the subject of headsails, avoid standing on a headsail which is lying on the deck. It is not good for either the sail or your own stability, since the slippery material will slide around under your feet and you will inevitably fall over.

Be prepared

Prepare all the sails for hoisting before you leave the berth. You may often see yachts, racing yachts especially, putting to sea from the marina or mooring with no headsail prepared, perhaps even with the boom cover still on. A cruising yacht skipper may be planning to motor some distance before making sail; racing skippers will certainly be waiting until shortly before the race start before selecting which of their many headsails to use – but their crews will then have the task of preparing the sail for hoisting while the yacht bucks around in a seaway, and they get wet. Being racing sailors they won't mind that – it's all part of the image. When cruising it is both more comfortable and better seamanship to have all the sails

ready for hoisting before heading out. You never know when the engine might pack up.

BELOW

Inevitably, bags, boxes of food and bottles of drink will have been brought on board and probably dumped on settees, the chart table and the galley worktops. These must be properly stowed before the yacht leaves her berth. It is too easy, in the excitement of getting away, to say 'oh, leave them for now; we can stow those as we go down the river' or whatever. But be warned: numberless vessels of all ages have suffered calamity from too hurried a rush to leave harbour before they were 'in all respects ready for sea', as the hallowed phrase has it. Your yacht may not founder because a box of groceries tumbles off a settee as she first heels to the breeze, but it is surprising what a mess it can make.

You may not have any gun ports or bow doors to close, but remember to check that any opening ports or windows in the topsides or cabin sides have been closed and secured, before someone winds up with a sodden bunk and the bilges are awash.

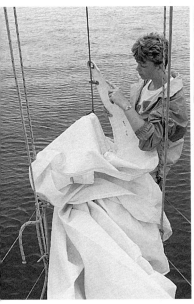 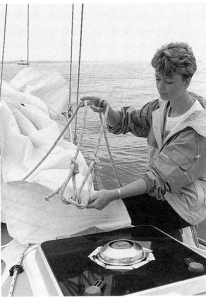 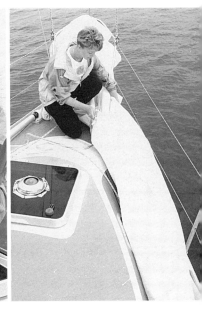

Attach all the hanks to the forestay . . . *Tie the sheets to the clew, using bowlines . . .* *And lash the sail to the rail.*

LEAVING THE BERTH

This is principally the skipper's problem, but as crew you will be expected to assist with letting go the mooring lines. You may also have to help 'walk' the yacht away from her berth, especially if she is in an awkward corner of a crowded marina, but since most cruising yachts these days have auxiliary motors you will probably drive away.

If you are leaving the permanent berth the mooring lines may well be left on the dock, to be picked up when you return. Otherwise you will take your lines with you. Bring them on board smartly. There are two reasons for this: it is sloppy and untidy to motor round with odd loops of line hanging over the rail, but more to the point there is a good chance that a line trailing in the water will quickly find its way around the propeller.

Even a small line will hook over the spinning propeller blade, jam the prop and stall the engine. If this happens there will not only be no way of motoring the boat forward, but there will also be no way of slowing it down save by running it into something.

By the same token, never leave fenders hanging over the side after you leave the berth.

↻ *Bring all the lines aboard as you leave.*

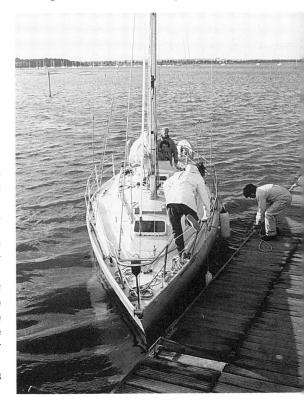

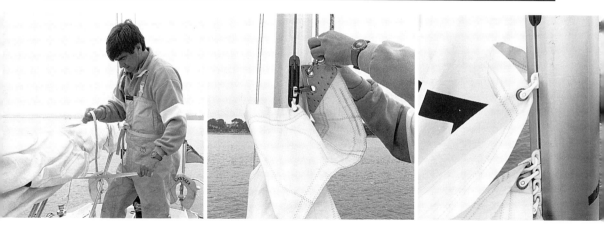

⌂ *Undo the mainsail ties . . .*   *Shackle the halyard to the head . . .*   *Check the luff slides . . .*

They look untidy and express less than total confidence in the abilities of the skipper. Inevitably, if they are needed to help get the boat away from her surroundings , they will be in the wrong place. If you think a fender or two may yet be needed, keep it handy and unattached, ready for whisking instantly to the likely point of impact.

Never, ever, try to act as a human fender yourself. Even a tiny yacht, or for that matter a dinghy, can snap a human bone like a cocktail stick.

SETTING SAIL

Once in open water the sails will be set, usually mainsail first. The golden rule before hoisting any sail is check everything twice, especially aloft, and leave attaching the halyard to last. With the boat jumping around and no weight on the halyard, if it is attached too early it will soon swing itself around something it should not be around, or swing itself off something it should be around, such as the turning sheave at the top of the mast.

Hoisting the mainsail

Attach the main halyard to the head of the sail, and thereafter tend it constantly, preferably by hoisting the sail immediately. Be sure to insert the luff of the sail in the mast track before hauling away.

The topping lift will take the weight of the mainboom until the sail is up and set. This is the line rigged from the end of the boom to the mast head. Someone must be tending the mainsheet, ready to ease it as the sail goes up; if this is not done, the wind in the sail will at the very least make hard work of hoisting it, and may well cause the sail to be pressed against some obstruction which may rip it.

You will usually have to turn the boat head to wind before hoisting the mainsail, but she can then be laid off onto her course before setting the headsail. Inevitably the engine will still be running, so inevitably any line – the tail of the halyard, for instance – that goes over the side will go round the prop.

Only when the sail is up and the halyard tensioned and secured should any of the other controls such as the sheet and boom vang be put under load.

Hoisting the headsail

It is usually easier and better to hoist and set the headsail with the yacht already sailing (or motor-sailing). That way the sail blows clear of the mast and the rigging as it goes up, and does not damage itself by flapping against them (or anyone still on the foredeck, who is likely to come off much the worse in any argument with a flogging sail and its associated rope and hardware).

Clip the hanks onto the forestay from the bottom up. Once the sail is fully hanked on, attach the halyard and haul away. Secure the halyard on its cleat, making sure it is well tensioned, and pull the sheet on to bring the sail under control. The less flogging the sail is

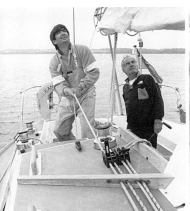

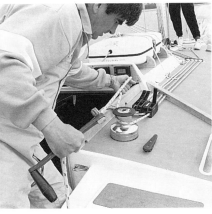

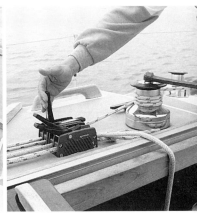

And haul away.   *Winch the halyard tight . . .*   *And jam it with the stopper.*

allowed to do, the better. Flogging and flapping are just about the worst things that can be allowed to happen to any sail: they break down the fibres and stitching of the sail, and shorten its life dramatically. Despite this you often see boats being handled with sails left to flog themselves to death against anything and everything. Sails are very expensive; perhaps if each came with a flogometer attached, where each crack of the sail rang up the price of a can of beer, crews would take more care of them.

Bliss

Once the sails are set, the engine can be switched off. There is a blissful moment when the stop lever is pulled, the engine dies, someone rushes to turn the key and stop that infernal hooter (the battery drain alarm, which sounds when the engine is switched on but not running), silence descends and the first hiss of a passing sea is heard unadulterated by mechanical sound. Nine times out of ten, someone in the crew will say: 'that's better'.

↻ Attach the halyard to the head of the headsail . . .   *And heave away on the halyard to haul the sail up the forestay.*   *Once the sail is up, sheet it in to stop it flapping.*

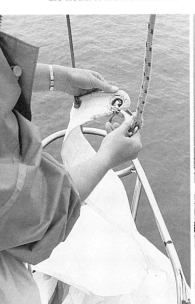

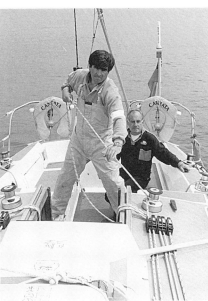

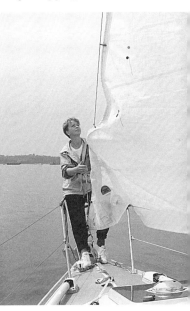

6 Sailing along

At last we are under sail, on passage for our first destination. The sails are our motive power, and will require careful attention. Were we racing, trimming the sails would be the constant and all-consuming task. Since we are cruising we want to have time to look around and do other things – but even so, life will go serenely only if the sails are properly trimmed and cared for.

A minimum of theory

The landlubber thinks that it is the wind blowing into the bellying sail which pushes the boat along. Needless to say, the landlubber is wrong. Unless you are running before the wind, it is the wind blowing *across* the sail which *pulls* the boat along. Once you have grasped this not-so-obvious notion, the whole art of sailing and sail trimming begins to open like a book.

As you look up into the curve of the sail, you can see how the wind does its work. As it arrives at the front edge of the sail (the luff), the wind bends to follow the sail's curve, flowing along the sail. The breeze on the outside of the curve has further to go to get to the trailing edge of the sail (the leech) than the breeze on the inside, so it has to travel faster. In doing so, a pressure difference is created, with the lower pressure on the outside of the sail, the higher pressure on the inside. To equalise the pressure the sail tries to move into that 'vacuum', and pulls the boat along with it. A physicist might explain things rather differently, and take a good deal longer, but if we keep this simple explanation in mind we can see how best to trim any sail for upwind sailing – that is, sailing towards the direction from which the wind is coming.

At its most simplistic, the more we can get the sail to curve, the more we bend the breeze blowing across it and the faster the boat will go. The sail should always be trimmed so that the luff lies along the path of the air blowing onto it. This effectively 'captures' the wind; then, the more we bend the wind with the sail, the more power we can extract from it.

↪ *The sail acts like a soft aircraft wing, bending the airflow to create 'lift'.*

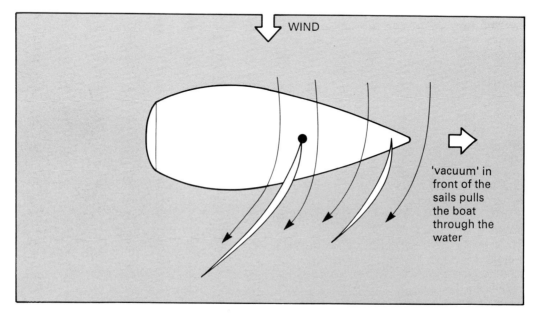

WIND

'vacuum' in front of the sails pulls the boat through the water

TRIMMING THE HEADSAIL: UPWIND

Since the sail is soft, it is actually quite easy to see when the luff is lined-up with the wind's direction because the whole sail takes up a nice curve. If the sail is let out too far the wind blows into the back part of the sail, not the inside face, and you can see that the very front part of the sail is filling from the wrong side. The sail must be pulled in a little bit to line up the luff correctly.

It is not so easy to tell if you have pulled it in too far, since the sail is still filling from the correct side. It is not working efficiently, but there is no visible evidence of this. So the trick is to let the sheet out a bit until the luff starts to flap, then pull it in an inch or two.

You will go a long way in sailing before you will find a better rule-of-thumb for sail-trimming than this:

> *Let it out until it starts to flap*
> *Then pull it in until it stops.*

Halyard tension

The other control affecting the shape of the headsail is the halyard. If it is too tight the halyard over-stretches the luff of the sail, but if it is too loose it leaves the luff saggy and baggy, preventing the sail from setting nicely and, in particular, seriously limiting the sail's ability to perform when sailing upwind.

Fortunately, it is easy to see when the halyard is not right. If it is too tight you will get a hard fold of cloth, a sort of double edge, running down the luff of the sail parallel to the forestay. If the halyard is too loose you will first see tiny pucker-lines radiating out and back into the sail from each of the hanks, then you will notice that the luffrope of the sail is curved between each of the hanks.

If the yacht has a grooved forestay rather than hanks, these pucker-lines will appear as horizontal folds, pulling aft across the sail.

In either case the halyard tension should be just enough to stretch the luff into a smooth line. The actual tension required will depend on the weight of wind in the sail: the more wind, the more tension is needed in the halyard.

Similarly, because sailing into the wind puts more pressure on the sails then sailing away

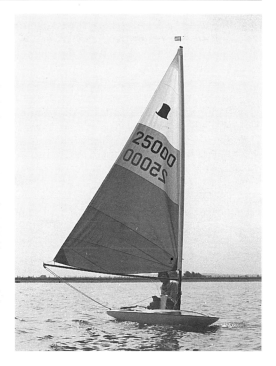

⌂ *The striped sail on this dinghy demonstrates what happens when you let the sail out too far.*
▽ *The effect of a loose halyard.*

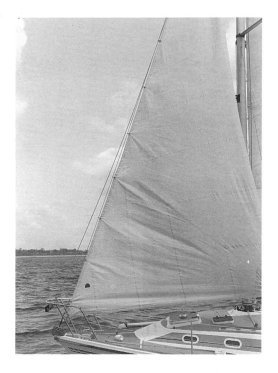

from the wind, you will need more halyard tension when sailing upwind.

Sheet lead position

This also affects the shape of the sail. Moving the lead aft increases the tension on the foot while at the same time decreasing tension in the leech; moving it forward does the opposite. To start with, the lead should be in the position which gives equal tension in leech and foot as the sheet is pulled in.

The sheet lead position is also used to alter the amount of twist in the headsail. Adjusting the lead to alter the twist allows the headsail to be set 'married' to the mainsail; if you look up the leech of the headsail, the line it takes should be parallel with the curve of the mainsail for as far as possible, until the point where the head of the headsail is attached to the mast.

Moving the sheet lead aft gives more twist in the sail; that is, it allows the top of the sail to blow further out than the bottom. Moving the sheet lead forward gives less twist.

▷ Here the sheet lead is well forward on its track to reduce twist in the headsail.
▷ The headsail leech of this racing yacht is perfectly 'married' to the curve of the main.

TRIMMING THE SAILS TOGETHER

Because the wind being bent round the headsail affects the mainsail, it is normal on any point of sailing to trim the headsail first, then trim the mainsail. Having done that you look at the headsail again, then at the mainsail, and so on . . .

Remember, the wind is never constant for long in either direction or strength, and every alteration of wind requires a corresponding alteration of the sails. Just how conscientiously you tend the sail trim is up to you and the skipper – but it is also a measure of how good a sailor you are. The yacht will only work as well as you allow her to work.

TRIMMING THE MAINSAIL – UPWIND

Much the same rules apply, except that since the mainsail foot is held rigid by the mainboom, the mainsail is usually less revealing than the headsail.

Even so the old adage about letting it out until it flaps applies, except that the flapping will initially be confined to ever-increasing backwinding along the luff (down the mast).

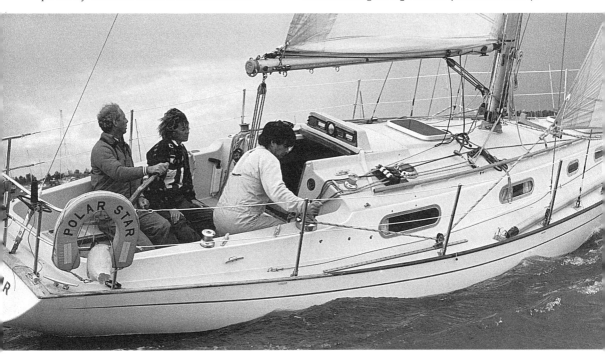

If the yacht has a burgee or wind indicator at her masthead you can apply another rough but surprisingly accurate rule of thumb by easing the mainsheet until the headboard at the top of the mainsail is lined up with the direction of the burgee.

The vang (kicking strap)

As the mainsheet is eased, the boom can go not only out but also up. The pressure of the wind in the sail will try to make it do just that, and the vang is there to prevent it.

We need to prevent the boom rising because as it does so the cloth in the sail goes slack, particularly at the leech, and this allows the sail to twist horribly. If the sail is twisted you cannot line it up properly with the wind angle, for when the bottom of the sail is properly aligned, the top is too far out and just flaps. To get the top right, you have to pull in the lower part of the sail much too far.

The vang or kicking strap – which may be a block and tackle or a rigid strut of some sort –

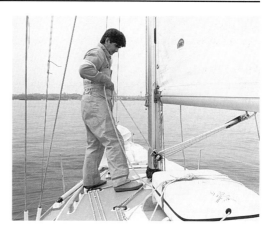

⌂ Tensioning the vang holds the boom down and reduces twist in the mainsail.

runs diagonally from the foot of the mast where it joins the deck to the underside of the boom, and holds the boom down. But it does more than this.

Adjusting the tension on the vang adjusts the shape of the mainsail outer edge, or leech. The more tension, the straighter or tighter the leech.

If the leech is too tight there will be too much belly in the sail and the whole sail will be choked; if the leech is too loose there will be too much twist in the sail and the yacht will be losing power.

A good rule of thumb for judging the correct amount of twist is to ease the vang until the top batten in the sail is parallel to the mainboom. If the sail has no battens, line up the boom with the leech of the sail about a quarter of the way down from the top.

Halyard and foot tension

Adjust the halyard tension as explained for the headsail. The foot tension is adjusted via the clew outhaul at the end of the boom, and works in exactly the same way.

Adjust both to suit the pressure of wind in the sail so that the tape which runs along both luff and foot appears smooth and taut, but not stretched.

One notable exception to this might be in very light winds, especially sailing downwind when you want the sails to be as full (to have as much belly) as possible. Then you might ease the foot and halyard tensions to just the point where wrinkles appear in the luff and foot tapes.

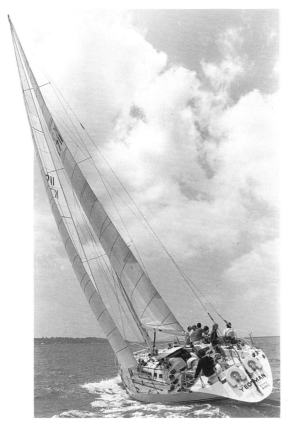

STEERING A COMPASS COURSE

You may think that steering the boat is the job of the skipper, but sooner or later everyone takes a turn. It is actually one of the easiest jobs on board, but it gives you a great sense of responsibility. You really feel in control of the boat – or you should.

When you take the helm for the first time try to get the feel of it by steering a little to port, then a little to starboard and back again. This will probably upset the sail trim, and you'll learn three things fast: the way the boat reacts to the helm, the way the sails react to minor course changes and the way the rest of the crew react to bad steering.

Once you have the feel of the boat you can settle down to steering the course. On a cruising boat the skipper will have worked out a course to steer, and the previous helmsman should tell you this when you take over. It will be a compass course, corrected for any magnetic anomalies in the ship's compass which should be somewhere on the bulkhead in front of you.

The average ship's compass is a fluid-filled bubble containing a revolving compass card marked in degrees. If the skipper asks you to steer 330 degrees you aim the boat so the 330-degree mark is aligned with the line on the bubble (the lubber line), and hold it there.

So much for the theory. In practice it's not immediately obvious which way to turn the boat, and in any case the compass card tends to swing around with every wave.

You can sort out the direction to steer by going into your port and starboard routine again, watching the compass as you do it. See how it swings off course as you move the tiller or wheel, and note the way you have to move the tiller or wheel to correct it. You should be able to work out a rule of thumb: to shift the compass card to the left, move the helm *this* way; to shift it to the right, move the helm *that* way. It may help to remember that the compass card stays still, and the boat revolves around it. If the boat has an electronic digital compass you will have to think slightly differently, and move the helm to make the numbers go up or down.

The problem of the swinging compass card is easily solved. Watch it for a bit. It will probably swing fairly consistently over, say, ten degrees. So if the course ordered is 330 degrees, make sure the card never swings beyond 325 or 335 degrees. The yacht's heading will be an average of the two – 330 degrees.

On some points of sailing it may be more important to steer by the sails, to keep them drawing or to prevent an accidental gybe. Fine, but watch the compass and tell the skipper the *actual* course you are having to sail. He can then update his plot, check for hazards and if necessary revise his navigation plan while you keep the boat going.

If you have real trouble keeping to the course, tell the skipper. He will need to know, so he can keep the navigation plot up to date. There's no shame in owning up, but keeping quiet could be catastrophic.

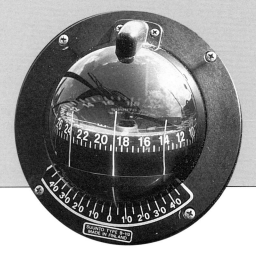

USING A HAND-BEARING COMPASS

A hand-bearing compass is designed for taking accurate visual bearings of landmarks, buoys and beacons, lights and other vessels. It has a revolving compass card instead of a needle, and a prism which shows the bearing when the compass is held up to your eye (or at arm's length, depending on the design). The prism usually has a notch in the top which you use like a gunsight, lining up the notch with the object and reading off the bearing displayed beneath.

You may be asked to take a single bearing of, say, a conspicuous building. The navigator will use this to work up a position plot. Alternatively, the skipper may ask you to take a series of bearings of your destination to see if the boat is being pushed off course by the tide. If the bearings are all the same you are staying on track.

Taking a series of bearings of an approaching vessel shows whether you are on a collision course. If the bearings change appreciably then all is well, but if they stay the same then you will probably have to take avoiding action.

When you align an object with the sight of the compass the figure reflected in the prism gives its bearing. If the bearing of another vessel stays constant you are on a collision course.

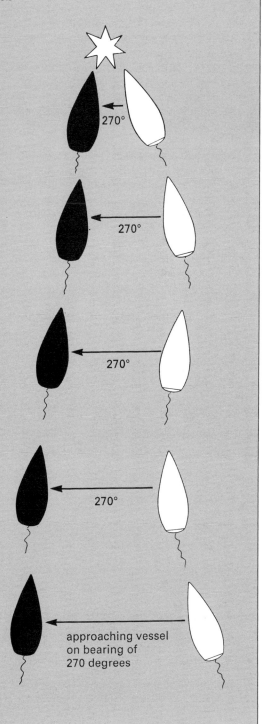

DOWNWIND SAILING

When the boat is steered directly downwind the mainsail tends to deflect all the wind from the headsail, which will not set properly. There are two ways of getting round this: you can either get rid of the headsail altogether and replace it with a spinnaker (see Chapter 10), or you can set the headsail on the other side of the boat, where it will not be blanketed by the main.

Poling out the headsail

Being soft-footed, the headsail will not stay full and drawing on the opposite side to the main without some assistance; it will always be collapsing in upon itself. The answer is to use a jib-boom to keep it spread.

The simplest jib-booms – usually called whisker-poles – have a spike at one end which pushes through the clew cringle of the headsail (the eye where the sheets are attached) and a

↳ *Rig the jib-boom and attach it to the fitting on the mast . . .*

fitting at the other to secure the inboard end to the mast. Often this is simply a Y-shaped crutch which presses against the front of the mast. To keep the whole arrangement in place you may need to adjust the position of the sheet lead.

The bigger the boat the more elaborate the gear. A yacht of say 35ft may carry a fully-rigged spinnaker pole for use as a jib-boom, complete with a sliding cup fitting on the mast.

Setting the jib-boom

1 With the headsail sheeted on the same side as the main, release the pole from its stowage and secure the foreguy or downhaul to the underside of the pole.
2 Take *plenty* of slack in the weather headsail sheet, for what comes later. Fit the weather sheet through the outboard end-fitting of the pole, so that the sheet runs freely.
3 Attach the topping lift. Lay the pole along the centre of the foredeck. Lift and fit the inboard end of the pole to the mast fitting.

Raise it level using the topping lift, controlling it with the foreguy . . .

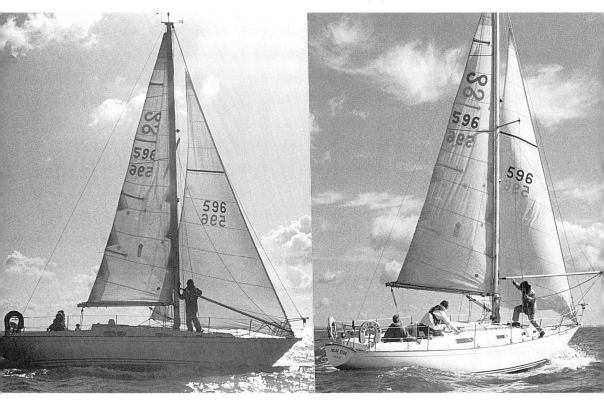

4 Lift the outboard end of the pole and support it while taking the weight on the topping lift.

5 The pole is now horizontal. It is also probably swinging about a good deal, banging against the forestay or headfoil. Control it with the foreguy, and work as quickly as possible to avoid damage to the boat, her gear or your own head.

6 In the cockpit, take up the slack on the weather sheet, and transfer the weight onto it while letting go the leeward sheet. Using the weather sheet, pull the sail across until it fills on the opposite side to the main. The closer to dead downwind the yacht can be sailed at this point, the easier this becomes. The pole may have to be pushed back along the sheet to bring the end of the pole and the clew of the sail close together.

7 Set the sail with the sheet, then tension the foreguy against the sheet so that the outboard end of the pole is held rigid and the pole does not swing around.

Using a whisker pole

1 Stand at the mast facing forwards, pole in one hand, weather jibsheet in the other. Fit the outboard end of the pole to the sail, making sure you are working on what will be the inboard side of the sail once it is boomed-out.

2 Keep the sail under control and attached to the pole by keeping tension on the weather sheet as you push the pole outboard and forward. Attach the inboard end of the pole to the mast.

3 Take up the tension on the weather sheet, through the weather-side fairlead and onto the winch.

Use the weather sheet to pull the sail across the boat to the end of the jib-boom . . .

Sheet in to make the sail fill, and tension the foreguy to hold the pole steady.

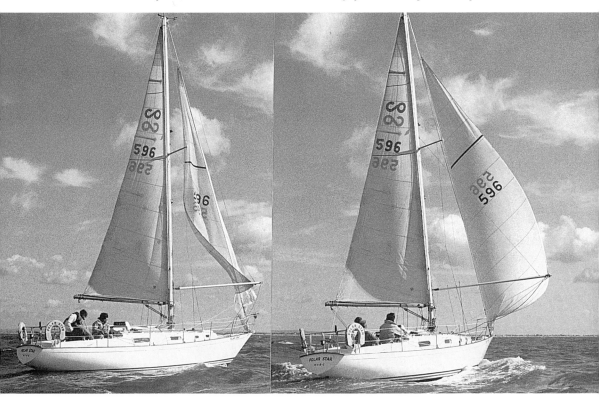

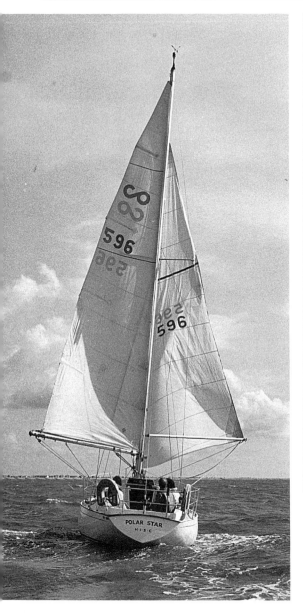

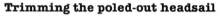

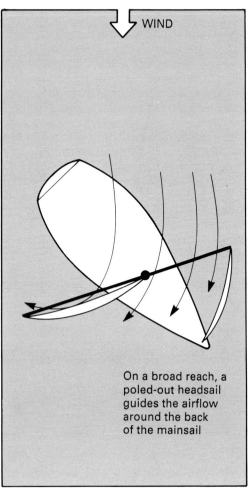

On a broad reach, a poled-out headsail guides the airflow around the back of the mainsail

⌂ *If you pole out the headsail on a reach, keep the pole in line with the main boom.*

Trimming the poled-out headsail

Dead downwind, the mainsail is let out as far as it will go, and the jib-boom brought back as far as the shrouds will allow.

A headsail poled out on the weather side is also very useful with the yacht on a broad reach. Here, the simple rule of thumb is that the mainboom and the jib-boom should be about in line, so trim the main until it is right and line up the pole with it. As you sheet in the mainboom you let the jib-boom forward.

The sheet lead

The further aft you bring the jib-boom, the further aft the sheet lead must be. With the boom squared right aft you may need to rig a separate sheet from a block at the aft end of the cockpit.

As the boom goes forward, so the sheet will fall foul across the shrouds, until you may see it actually start to bend the weather shroud. You should now think in terms of rigging a special reaching sheet *inside* the shroud – but by the time you get to this point of sailing you will probably find that the headsail sets perfectly well on the same side as the mainsail, so the jib-boom may be taken off.

Unshipping the jib boom

1 Set the boat on a course near dead down-wind. This is to transfer the weight of the sail to the leeward-side sheet, by taking in on that sheet and releasing the weather sheet. If this is attempted with the boat on a reach, all that happens is that as the weather sheet is eased the pole goes forward until it is on the forestay; as the new sheet is taken in, it has to drag the sail back across the forestay, which is bad for the sail.

2 With the sail transferred to the other sheet, put the boat back on a reach to stop the boom swinging around. Ease the topping-lift to lower the outboard end of the pole into the pulpit.

3 Release the weather sheet from the outboard end of the pole. Release the topping lift and take the inboard end of the pole off the mast. Stow the pole and tighten up the foreguy, if it is normally left attached to the pole.

4 Make sure the weather sheet is clear of the stowed pole, or on top of it, and that all is cleared away ready to tack.

RIGGING A MAIN PREVENTER

When you are running before the breeze, perhaps the greatest danger is that the yacht might stray off course far enough to allow the wind to get into the back of the mainsail, blowing it suddenly and violently across the boat in an accidental gybe. The dangers of something as solid and heavy as the mainboom scything across the deck at great speed hardly need to be dwelt upon; the accidental gybe is probably the commonest and most dangerous accident which can happen on board.

Peace of mind is assured by rigging a preventer (a very literal and descriptive name), in the form of a block and tackle from somewhere near the outboard end of the boom down to a block secured near the bow. Just how the preventer is rigged depends on the fittings available on the boat, but the preventer should be long enough to allow the boom to be eased right across the boat if necessary.

A handy-billy (see Chapter 3) with snap shackles at either end and a jamming cleat incorporated with the lower block makes an ideal preventer. It is quick and easy to use, powerful enough to hold the boom out if the

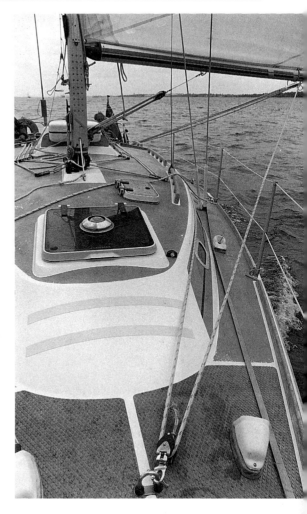

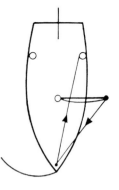

A preventer holds the boom out on the run and stops it sweeping across the deck in an accidental gybe. One way of rigging one is to run a long line from the boom end, through a block on the foredeck and back to a spare sheet winch.

mainsail does backfill, and can be quickly removed and re-rigged on the other side when the times comes to gybe on purpose.

NIGHT SAILING

Your first sail will probably be a short hop from port to port, with the sun sparkling on the water, the more comely members of the crew draped about the yacht in flimsy attire and the champagne cooling nicely in the fridge. This, of course, is what sailing is all about.

But some skippers get other ideas. They want to go on long trips that involve sailing overnight, when all sensible people are asleep. A skipper planning such a trip is apt to find himself short of crew at the critical moment; he will approach you with tall tales of foreign shores and the romance of the sea, and before you know it you have signed on. So you'll need to know something about night sailing.

Actually, it *can* be quite romantic. Most people who go cruising would agree that some of the best, most memorable moments occur at night, when the yacht is sailing well, half the crew are asleep and you and your watch companion are alone in the cockpit, swapping stories, guiding the ship over the waves and waiting for the first gleam of the landfall light.

Watch systems

During a day passage everyone is on deck all the time, unless they are preparing lunch, but at night you all need your sleep – including the skipper. The only way to manage this and still work the boat is to arrange a rota, or a watch system.

Watch systems vary depending on the skipper, the number of crew and the weather conditions. A normal night watch consists of two or three hours on deck, four to six hours below, then another two to three on deck. If there is only enough crew for two 'shifts' you may find your sleeping time halved, and watch times tend to get shorter as the weather deteriorates. On long passages the watch system is carried on through the day as well, but normally with a longer turnover time.

Organising the watch is the skipper's job, and he may change it half-way through the voyage. All you have to do is fit in with it.

Sleeping in short stretches does not come easily to the average person accustomed to eight hours in a comfortable bed. If you have been pulling your weight on deck you should have no trouble dropping off, but being woken

up four hours later can be hard to take. On any civilised boat the shock is cushioned by rousing the next watch with a hot drink and allowing some waking-up time of 15 minutes or so. Once you are up and awake you return the courtesy by putting the kettle on for those coming off watch, and then go up on deck to relieve them. Make sure you turn up on time; being late on watch is just about the worst crime you can commit, and nothing will turn a pleasant cruise sour more quickly.

On deck

The first thing you do as you climb the companionway steps is clip on. You should be wearing your safety harness; clip its safety line to the fitting in the cockpit, if necessary by passing it to someone who is already there, before you emerge. If you stumble as you climb out and pitch over the leeward guardrails the harness line will save you, but if you are not clipped on you will vanish in the dark.

Always clip on at night. A person overboard during the day is bad enough, but at night it is certain catastrophe. Make sure it can't happen. If you have to go forward to work on a headsail transfer the clip to the jackstay running along the side deck *before* you leave the cockpit, and pull the line after you as you move forward, being careful not to get it tangled in the rigging.

If there are only two of you on watch you may have to take a turn at the helm. This will probably be a matter of steering a compass course. The compass will be illuminated so you can see it, but try not to stare at it all the time. You can become mesmerised by the compass and ignore everything else; what's more the light in the compass could ruin your night vision. You should avoid using any lights on deck for the same reason.

Keep a good look-out. There is a temptation to scan the horizon, check there are no lights nearby and then settle back to enjoy a good conversation, but in busy waters there is always a risk of running into an unlit hazard such as a chunk of deck cargo that has fallen off a freighter. It will probably never happen, but you should be aware of the possibility.

Watch for other vessels on a collision course with you. They should be carrying lights, and on a dark night this is all you will see. Judging

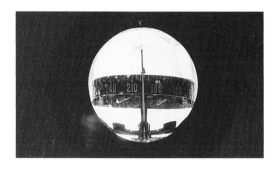

⟳ *Don't stare at the compass; it can blind you.*

the course of another vessel from its lights alone is a tricky business; do not rely on a casual glance, but use a hand-bearing compass to determine the risk of collision (see page 45).

If you consider that there might be a danger of collision, rouse the skipper. Indeed, if you are unsure about anything you see, or think that the yacht is carrying too much sail, or the tiller comes off in your hand – rouse the skipper. He would much prefer that you got him up for no good reason than let him sleep on while his boat heads into trouble. If he gives you a hard time about it, he's a poor skipper.

Normally the skipper will give you some instructions before turning in: the course to steer, lighthouses to watch for, the things you can do without waking him. He may even write it down. He will certainly want you to keep the ship's log up to date; if he fails to mention this, then ask. A proper record of the course steered, distance run and any observations

made is essential to his navigation. Remember: if he gets lost, you are lost too.

Back down below

When your time is up, go below. Don't be tempted to extend your watch just because you've got into the groove. If you are having a good time it's bad manners to deprive others of the pleasure. If the weather is bad you may feel inclined to let the next watch sleep in for a bit, but they will then feel impelled to do the same for the watch following. Before you know it the whole system has broken down.

When you go below, rouse the next watch, put the kettle on and make them something to drink. Then leave them to it. When they emerge on deck (they may need a little coaxing) help them clip on and fill them in on any developments. Hang around for a bit while they get themselves sorted, then go below and stay there.

If the boat is lurching around and you suffer from seasickness, get horizontal as soon as possible. Don't bother to undress – just crash out in the bunk. If you spend more than one night at sea this could get a bit unsavoury, but hopefully the second night will be calmer. In heavy weather you will need a leeboard to stop you falling out, but if you are 'hot-bunking' the board will already be fitted. Slip your mind out of gear and go to sleep. When you wake it will be morning, the sun will be sparkling on the water and someone will be crashing around in the galley looking for the champagne.

⟳ *A leeboard will keep you in your bunk during your watch below.*

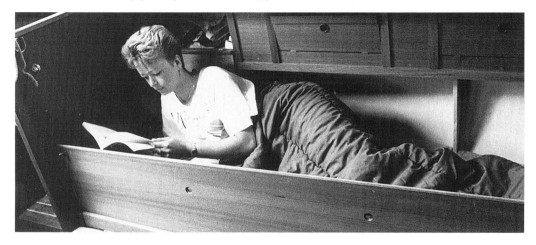

7 Tacking and gybing

Under power you can steer in any direction you like by simply turning the wheel, but when you are sailing it is not so easy. As you change the yacht's heading relative to the wind you have to adjust the sails to keep them working properly – and if you try to sail directly into the wind the sails will not work at all. If you change direction so radically that the wind blows from the other side of the boat you will have to move the whole rig to the other side too, in a controlled fashion. When sailing upwind this is called tacking; when sailing downwind it is known as gybing. Both manoeuvres can be quite complex, depending on the yacht, but they are an essential part of working the boat.

TACKING

When you are sailing upwind the sails have to be curved to generate power. Because each sail is flexible it will only take up the necessary curve if just one side is presented to the wind. If the wind is allowed to affect both sides of the sail it simply flutters like a flag.

In practice, reducing the angle between the sail and the wind direction to anything much less than 40 degrees presents the sail at too acute an angle to the wind, and it starts to flap in exactly the same way as a sail that is trimmed out too far. It stops pulling the boat through the water, and as a result it is impossible to make headway with the boat heading directly into the wind.

If you want to travel in that direction you have to sail at the closest angle you can with the wind on one side, then turn and do the same with the wind at the same angle on the other side, zig-zagging back and forth but getting ever nearer your destination.

◊ *As the yacht tacks through the eye of the wind the sails backfill, then flutter uselessly like flags before filling on the other side of the boat.*

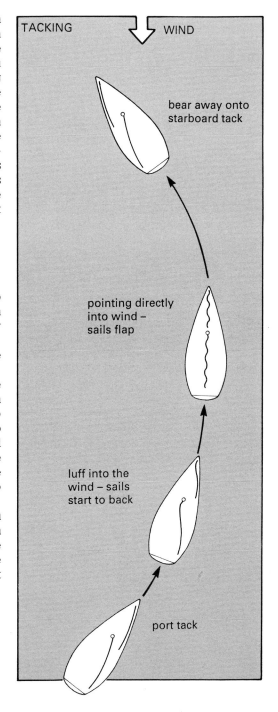

TACKING   WIND

bear away onto
starboard tack

pointing directly
into wind –
sails flap

luff into the
wind – sails
start to back

port tack

This zig-zagging is called beating, but the actual action of turning the yacht through the wind's eye is called tacking. When the yacht is beating with the wind blowing from the port side it is said to be on port tack; if it is beating with the wind blowing from the starboard side it is on starboard tack.

↻ *A 'square' course as sailed in a yacht, beating into the wind and gybing downwind.*

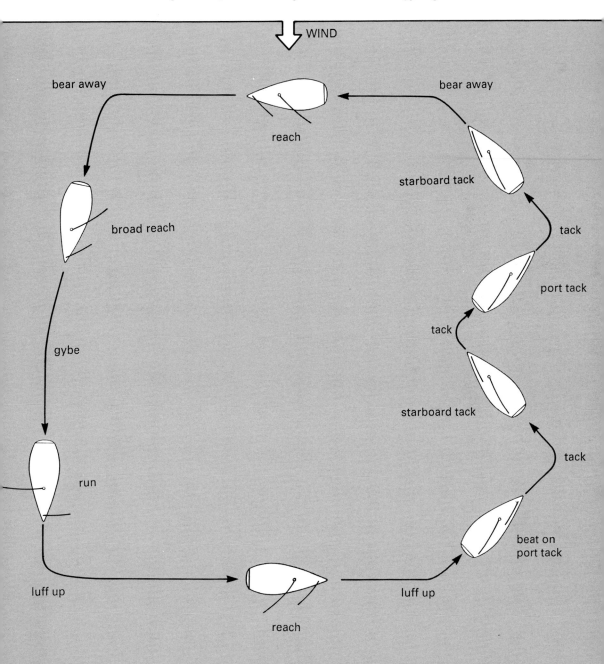

WHICH SIDE?

If you are new to sailing you may be confused by the terms port and starboard, windward and leeward.

Port and starboard

Essentially, port and starboard mean left and right. (If in doubt, remember that port has the same number of letters as left.) But they are not quite the same thing. The port side of the boat is always the left-hand side *when you are facing forward* – so if you are facing aft (towards the back of the boat) the port side of the yacht will be on your right. The principle is the same as the nearside and offside of a car.

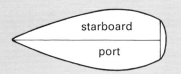

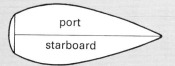

Windward and leeward

The windward or weather side of a boat or sail is the side facing the wind, while the leeward side – pronounced looward – is the side facing away from the wind. If the yacht is heeling over it will nearly always be heeling to leeward, so leeward is the downhill, wet side.

   If the yacht is running downwind the wind is coming directly over the stern, so strictly speaking there is no windward or leeward side. Despite this the terms are still used, with the position of the main boom indicating the leeward side.

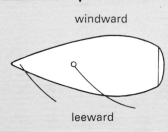

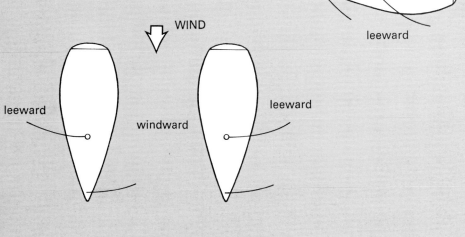

On board

The trick is to let the yacht and the wind do the work. As the helmsman puts the helm down the crew releases the old headsail sheet, and as the boat turns through the wind the slack on the new headsail sheet is hauled in. As she steadies up on the new course the wind itself should blow the headsail clear of the forward rigging. This is the moment to haul hard on the new sheet, winching the sail home before there is any real weight of wind in it.

Good timing is vital – and it helps to have a sensitive helmsman who sails the boat through the tack, rather than just flinging her round as fast as he can. In particular, a good helmsman will slow the turn in its final moments, just as the headsail blows free of the shrouds, to give the crew the chance to sheet it home.

If the sail fills before it is fully sheeted, life can be made easier by sailing slightly off the wind for a moment to let the boat gather way, and then getting the helmsman to steer close to the wind to take the weight of wind out of the sail while the crew bring home the final foot or so of sheet. Although unthinkable to the racing man, this is infinitely less wearisome than struggling over the winch in the lee side of a well-heeled cockpit, and in reality the yacht loses very little ground.

Tacking step-by-step

1 Prepare for the tack by hauling in the slack on the loose headsail sheet on the weather side; load the sheet on to the winch, using a maximum of three turns. Check that the leeward sheet is not full of kinks and snags, but is free to run.

2 Keeping tension on the tail (so as not to let the turns slip), take the sheet off the cleat. Hold the sheet on the winch by pressing the flat of your hand against the turns on the drum.

3 As the helm goes down, hold on to the sheet until the headsail starts to backfill at the luff, then quickly fling the turns off the winch. Do this by holding the tail about two feet from the winch, with the sheet at a slightly rising angle; ease the tension until the turns begin to slip, then twirl the sheet off the winch from above, rather as if you were trying to lassoo the winch – but in reverse. With most modern winches you will be twirling anti-clockwise, since the winch turns clockwise. Once the sheet is off

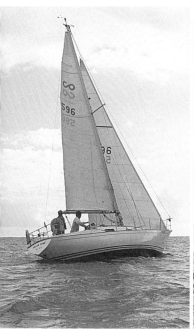

↻ From starboard tack, steer into the wind . . .

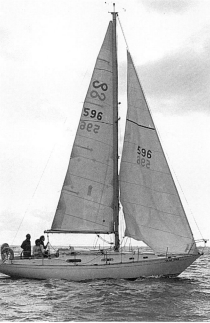

The sails flap as the boat heads directly upwind . . .

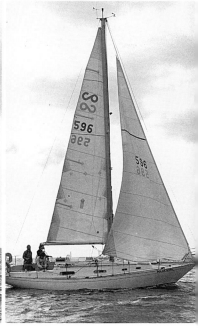

Then fill on the other side as she firms up on port tack.

the winch make sure the whole sheet is free to run through the turning block.

4 Take in the new sheet on its winch, pulling fast to keep the sheet taut and prevent riding turns. Put on extra turns as soon as it becomes difficult to take in the sheet by hand. Insert the handle and start winching.

5 Finally, remove the handle from the winch and replace it in its pocket, then load the new weather winch ready for the next tack. Apart from anything else, this is a good way of keeping the loose sheet secure.

If the yacht has running backstays prepare by bringing in the slack of the new runner and loading the tail onto the winch. Bring in only the slack; the runner has to be left soft to accommodate the belly of the mainsail until the yacht goes into the tack. As the yacht comes upright, wind in the new runner so that you have it fully home just as the yacht is head to wind. Let go the old backstay as soon as the yacht goes through head-to-wind, so that the mainsail can take up its proper shape without pressing against the backstay.

Common faults

● *Not keeping tension on the tail as you take it off the cleat.* The load on the sheet immediately starts to pull it off the winch. As the turns tighten the sheet locks up again, but you have lost several inches of sheet and now the sail is not drawing properly. Not taking care at this stage can be dangerous, especially if you are caught so unawares the sheet rips out of your hand and lets go completely. Flailing ropes are surprisingly hard when they hit you on the hands or in the face.

● *Letting go the old sheet too early, with wind still in the sail.* Again, this is potentially dangerous. Even if no one gets hurt, the yacht suddenly loses power just when she needs it to help her into the wind. One bad wave could stop her completely.

● *Letting go too late.* The sail backfills completely, stopping the yacht and then spinning her head off too quickly on the other tack, causing difficulty getting the new sheet in. You risk damaging the sail as it first presses against the rigging and then drags across to the other side.

● *Not clearing the out-going sheet.* There is a tendency for the rope to kink where it has been turned round the winch drum. Unless cleared these links snag in the turning block, stopping the sheet going out and hanging-up the headsail so that it cannot come across.

● *Sheeting in too early.* You pull the sail across too soon, so it backfills on the new side and quite possibly prevents the yacht from tacking altogether. Even if the bow is through the eye of the wind, sheeting in too fast pulls the leech of the sail tightly against the forward side of the shrouds and spreaders, increasing chafe and possibly causing the sail to catch and maybe tear.

● *Sheeting in too slowly, or too late.* You give yourself a lot of extra work, since you have to sheet-in the sail when it is already full of wind.

Common faults: running backstays

● *Pulling the new runner on too hard, too soon.* This distorts and chafes the back of the mainsail.
● *Not getting the new runner on quickly enough.* The top of the mast (which the running back-

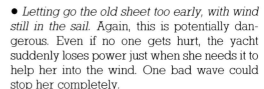

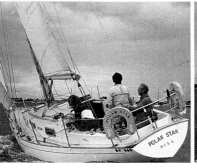
↻ *Prepare to release the old headsail sheet . . .*

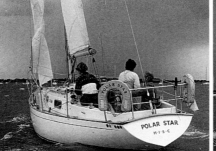
Let the sheet slip, then fling it off the winch as the sail flaps . . .

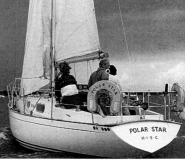
And take in the new sheet on its winch.

stay is there to support) is already leaning over to leeward. It is hard work to winch it back, and if you have no runner winches but use only tackle, you may not be able to set the runner properly.

• *Not getting the old runner off quickly enough.* The new stay cannot be set up properly because it is working against the old one. As it fills the mainsail presses against the old runner, ruining the set of the sail.

• *Leaving the leeward runner on its winch.* This is very dangerous, since with the leeward runner set up, or partly so, the mainsail cannot be eased; this makes it difficult or even impossible for the yacht to alter course to leeward. If you expect to tack again soon you can pre-turn the runner tail on the winch, ready for the tack. If you expect to be on the new tack for some time, take the leeward runner right forward and secure it at the shrouds to prevent chafe on the back of the mainsail. This is especially important on larger boats where the running backstay arrangement incorporates heavy blocks which would otherwise swing around dangerously.

GYBING

Gybing is rather like tacking, but the yacht turns with her stern towards the wind direction instead of her bow. The wind holds the mainsail on the 'old' side until the last minute, then gets behind it and may flip it abruptly – even violently – to the new side. This can be an alarming experience, and as a result most sailors treat gybing with a good deal of respect.

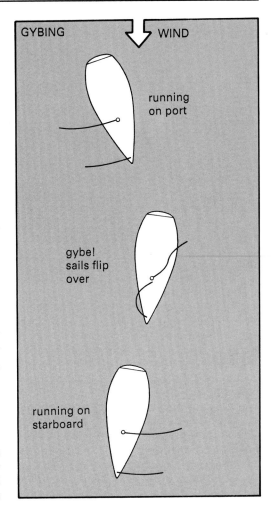

GYBING   WIND

running on port

gybe! sails flip over

running on starboard

⌒ *In a gybe, the sails are flicked to the other side of the boat by the pressure of wind blowing from behind.*

As the mainsail and boom swing across the boat . . .

Keep hauling in the new sheet until it is tight . . .

Then put extra turns on the winch and winch it home.

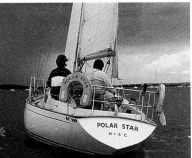

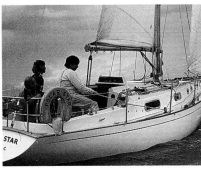

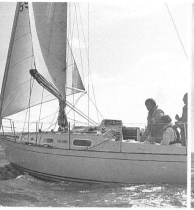

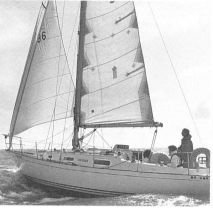

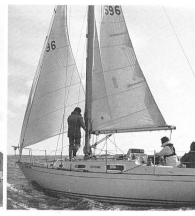

⌂ *Before the gybe, the mainsail is right out to port.*

Haul in the mainsheet through the blocks to bring the sail across . . .

And let it run out to fill on the new side.

The secret is – as always – to prepare beforehand and then take the manoeuvre itself gently but firmly. The helmsman needs to 'steer small', altering course just enough to bring the wind from one corner of the transom (the back of the boat) to the other as the mainsail is brought over the boat by hauling the mainsheet across.

In all but the very lightest breezes, always work the mainsheet through all its blocks; do not be tempted simply to grab the whole mainsheet tackle and heave that across. If anything goes wrong you stand a good chance of having your arm pulled out at the roots, and you will never be able to control or hold the mainsail once it has come across the boat and filled with wind on the other side.

Gybing the mainsail

1 If there is a traveller, centre the slider in the middle of the track.

2 Bring in the mainsheet *through the blocks*, not by grabbing the complete mainsheet and trying to pull the whole lot across.

3 As the mainsail comes to the centreline, the helmsman steers first dead downwind, then continues the turn. Help the boom across with a firm shove just as the wind goes into the back of the sail to blow it across, then let the mainsheet run. Because you close-hauled the sheet through the blocks, it must run out through them again and their friction acts as a brake, cushioning the boom's swing but letting the sail out fully and unhindered. If the sail should hang up just after the gybe the pressure in it

⌂ *To gybe the headsail, first raise the pole on the mast . . .*

Then lower the outboard end and release the sheet.

Swing the pole under the forestay and clip in the new sheet . . .

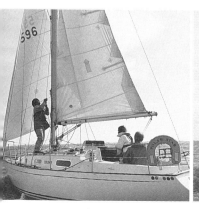

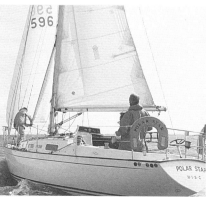

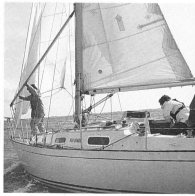

will try to turn the boat sharply up into the wind; with the rudder already turning the boat in that direction, she rounds up violently.

4 The helmsman should steer so as to stop the turn as soon as the boom comes across, reversing the helm to steer dead downwind again. 'Keep the boat under the rig' is the apt and expressive good advice.

The headsail

Gybe the mainsail first, then the headsail. With a simple whisker pole, you simply unship the pole, move the headsail across and re-rig the pole.

If you are using a spinnaker pole as a jib-boom life is a little more complex, because you do not want to manhandle the heavy pole more than you have to. The best way to gybe the pole is to leave the inboard end on the mast, unrig the sheet at the outboard end, swing the pole through underneath the forestay and re-rig it all on the other side. To get the pole under the forestay, lower the outboard end and, if necessary, raise the inboard end. The whole process is called dipping the pole.

1 Raise the inboard end of the pole on its slider track on the front of the mast, or reset the inboard end at its highest possible position if the boat only has fixed-position pole fittings.

2 Ease the sheet to let the pole go forward to the forestay and control the pole's tendency to swing with the foreguy or downhaul. Lower the outboard end of the pole on the topping lift, and at the same time release the sheet from the pole end by tripping the plunger.

3 Swing the pole under the forestay, catch the loose headsail sheet and fit it into the pole end, making sure the part of the sheet nearest the sail is on the forward side of the pole so the sheet runs the right way once the pole is up and the sail is boomed out again.

4 Raise the pole on the topping lift, lower the inboard end, sheet the sail on the new side and re-set the foreguy.

Running backstays

As the mainsail sheet is close-hauled, so the new running backstay is pulled on. Pause just before the gybe itself to let off and hold in hand the old runner, then release it as the boom starts across.

It is vital to get the old runner right off, and quickly. Otherwise the boom crashes against it and can travel no further. In heavy winds this might break the boom; certainly it will make the yacht round-up violently and heel right over under the press of mainsail – which cannot be released until the leeward runner is let go.

A common fault is not releasing the old runner quickly enough, or far enough. Because the running backstays are all that prevent the mast toppling over the bow, there is a natural fear that carelessness will lose the rig. True enough, but remember that when the mainsail is centred with the sheet it also holds up the mast (which is another reason for close-hauling the sheet through the blocks, rather than just flinging everything across the boat). As long as the new runner is pulled on and secured, even if it is not fully tensioned, the mast will be safe.

Pull the sail across using the new sheet . . .

Lower the inboard end of the pole until it is horizontal . . .

And sheet in the sail until it sets properly.

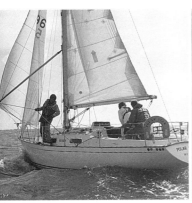
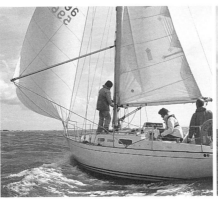
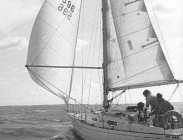

8 Lowering sails

As you get near your destination the skipper will want to get the sails down in good time and continue under engine. The first sail to come off will usually be the headsail. You need to be able to bring the sail down under control, prevent it (or its sheets) going over the side into the water, and then either get it quickly secured to leave the deck clear, or take it off altogether.

LOWERING THE HEADSAIL

Ease the sheet, but do not let it fly: this would simply allow the sail to flog around, possibly hitting someone (maybe you) in the face. Ease the sheet just enough to take the strain off the forestay, so that when the halyard is released

the sail comes down easily. This is particularly important if you are having to do the whole job by yourself.

If there is someone in the bow to gather the sail, uncleat the halyard and let it run, keeping it under control. If you have to deal with both halyard and sail yourself, make sure that the halyard is free to run right out as far as the stopper knot in the end. You can do this either by coiling it in big, loose coils which you then dump on the deck *with the loose end on the bottom* or by flaking it down in long parallel loops (see Chapter 11). Let the halyard go, and move smartly into the bow to gather the sail and stop it going overboard.

Pull the sail down the forestay, undo the halyard and clip it to the pulpit or top guardrail (it will slide back as far as the first stanchion, but

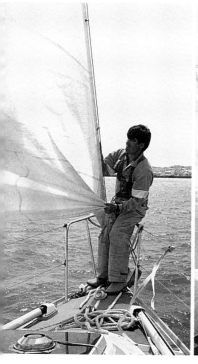
↷ *With the halyard released, prepare to gather the sail.*

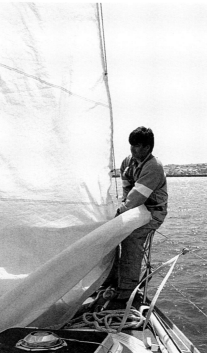
Gather it in loose folds on the foredeck as it comes down . . .

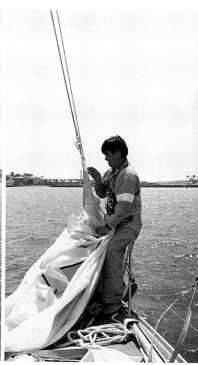
And unshackle the halyard from the cringle.

that does not matter). If the yacht has a headfoil with a luff groove, the whole sail is now attached only by the tack and the clew; if she has forestay hanks the sail is more secure, but either way it should be quickly lashed to the upper guard-rail with a sail tie. Pass the tie around the sail and over the rail, gathering the sail clear of the deck so it will not get in the way or get walked on.

For a short stay, you can simply lash the sail to the guardrail with a couple of ties and haul the sheet taut again. For an overnight stay you will either want to bag it and leave it hanked on and ready to go, or remove it altogether. Bagging a sail on the forestay is covered in Chapter 9. This is a neater method for a harbour stow, which has the twin advantages of inflicting less crumple damage on the sail and taking up much less room.

Bagging a harbour stow

Folding and bagging a sail on the foredeck is a job for two. One person takes the luff, the other the leech; the one at the luff is in the bow, facing aft, while the one at the leech stands by the mast inside the shrouds, facing forward.

Find the head, put that at one side, then follow down the luff piling the sail loosely on the head; this eventually leaves you with the foot of the sail stretched between you.

Keep a hand on each cringle (eyelet), and fold the round edge of the foot of the sail back over itself to give a straight fold between the cringles. Then take an arm's length of luff or leech with the other hand and fold it over so that the fold lies on top of the stretched foot. Pull the fold taut, smooth out any wrinkles and hold the folded edge under your knee. Take the next fold, pull it down – luff and leech together – to the foot, and so on.

Keep the luff folds aligned. Because the sail is triangular, this means that the leech folds work their way towards the luff and the person working the leech has to come with them, taking care not to skid on the folds of slippery cloth.

Eventually, you have the sail in flat concertina folds with the luff rope lying along itself and the head and tack cringles together.

Shackle the halyard to the rail to stow it.	*Grab a handful of sail ties (these are kept tied to the rail) . . .*	*And use them to secure the sail to the rail.*

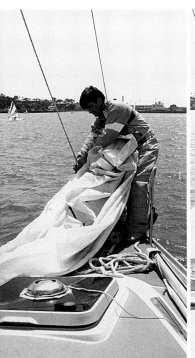 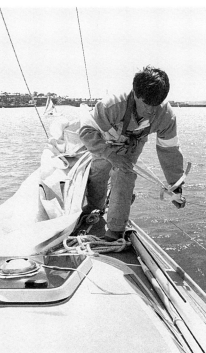 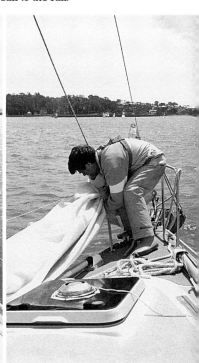

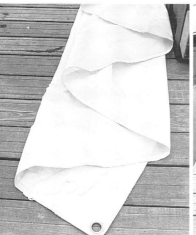
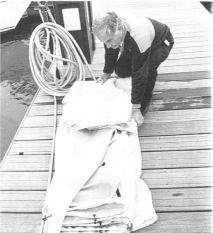
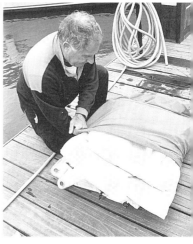

⤺ *For a harbour stow, flake the sail in concertina folds . . .*

Fold the bundle end to end, and keep on folding . . .

Until you can fit the result in the sail bag.

Bring the clew of the sail up to join the other corners, doubling the folded sail over lengthwise. Fold the doubled-over sail up towards the luff, using folds which will fit into the opened bag.

STOWING THE MAINSAIL

If there is any weight in the breeze you will have to turn the yacht into the wind before the mainsail comes down, or you will be left dragging the sail across the spreaders and rigging – assuming you can get it down the luff track at all. If the topping lift has been taken off the boom end while sailing, put it back.

Ease the vang and the mainsheet, then take the weight of the boom on the topping lift and raise it to a convenient working height. Let go the halyard, bring the sail down and immediately tension the mainsheet against the topping lift. This will hold the boom steady while you work at stowing the sail.

If the mast has a simple luff groove which takes the luff-rope of the sail the luff will fall all over the deck as the sail comes down. If the yacht is blessed with captive slides that fit into the groove or track the luff will remain captive – but the sail will bunch up on the mast above the gooseneck.

Take off the halyard as soon as you have the head at deck level; clip it out of the way.

⤺ *For a mainsail harbour stow drop the sail . . .*

Make concertina folds at the mast end . . .

While pulling them tight at the boom end.

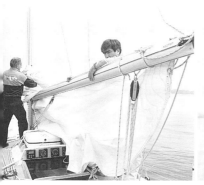
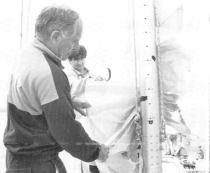
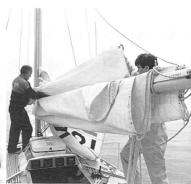

You may initially have to do a quick stow, leaving the neater harbour stow until there is more time (on some boats the quick stow *is* the harbour stow, making life as lazy for the crew as it is tough on the sails).

Quick stow

Arm yourself with a handful of sail ties and pull the main down, letting all the cloth fall on one side of the boom. If the luff of the sail is captive on the mast work up the leech from the aft end, pulling as much of the sail aft as you can.

Reach over the boom from the clear side and grab the leech and lower part of the sail at roughly one third of the height of the sail to form a bag into which the rest of the sail can be turned.

Holding the lower part of the sail away from the boom, tumble the upper part into the bag, then roll the sail in towards the boom, grabbing the lowest part of the roll and bringing that up over itself to form another roll. Then roll the sail in on itself as tightly as possible.

Ideally, tighten the roll down so that the very lower part of the sail forms a tight cover for the rest of the sail inside it. Secure it alongside or better still on top of the boom with the sail ties.

Take care to keep the leech pulled aft as you roll; this prevents the sail bunching at the mast end, and ensures that the battens in the sail lie flat along the boom and do not get broken as you try to roll them up with the sail.

If the luff is not captive on the mast you cannot pull the leech aft since the whole sail would come with it. Instead, you have to pull the leech and luff against each other to smooth out the

sail. It is, of course, much easier to roll the sail into itself if the luff is free.

Harbour stow

A proper harbour stow is both tidier-looking and better for the sail than bundling it up and leaving it there, creases and all.

The idea is to fold the sail back and forth across the boom so that it lies on top of the boom, with the folds draped to an even depth either side. There must be sufficient material either side to stop the whole lot sliding off the boom, but the folds must not be so deep that the mainsail cover cannot wholly cover the sail.

The more hands on this job, the easier it is.

If the sail comes right off the mast, the procedure is straightforward. Dump all the sail off to one side of the boom. One person then takes the luff, another the leech, and the rest deploy themselves along the boom to hold the partly folded sail and stop it slipping off – which it will try to do with wilful persistence.

Take about four feet of luff and a corresponding fold of leech, pull them taut against each other and then pull them both together back up over the boom, leaving about two feet on either side. Naturally the bigger the boat, the bigger the sail – and the bigger the folds. This first fold is crucial and lays the foundation for the whole stow; take time to get it right.

Carry on folding back and forth, pulling the cloth tight at each fold by holding the luff and pulling aft on the leech at the corresponding point.

Keep the luff together up at the gooseneck end; this means that the leech gradually works

The folds work their way gradually up the boom.

Secure the sail to the boom with the sail ties . . .

Then tighten everything up for a neat finish.

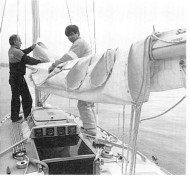
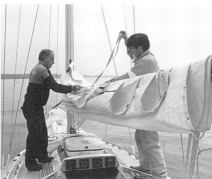
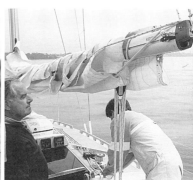

forward along the boom and has to be held in place by those helping in the middle. Stop after three or four folds and put a sail tie on the aft end to prevent the whole lot slipping off the boom when you have the job almost done.

If you are leaving the reefing lines in place, pull them through the boom at this stage until they are just taut; they will help keep the sail secure, and you will avoid the problem of trying to find somewhere to tuck them.

Carry on folding until you are left with just the head and enough cloth to go round the whole sail once. Pass the headboard under the boom and back up to lie on top of the folded sail. Pass the final sail tie through the cringle of the headboard to keep everything secure.

If the sail luff is held captive on the mast by its slides the sail is folded the same way; it is just a little more awkward.

Dump all the leech and as much of the sail as will go to one side of the boom. Open the gate on the mast track and drop off the lowest two slides; then close the gate and push the remaining slides and sail up the mast a little way so you can get at the gooseneck (the boom pivot).

↪ *You can make a seamanlike job of coiling the halyards by looping them over a winch.*

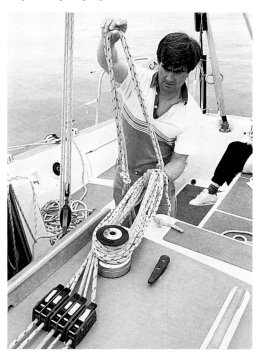

Pull the first fold through to one side, so the lowest slide is at the point of the first fold. Pull the luff and corresponding section of leech back across the boom until the next slide forms the point of the second fold. Holding the luff, pull back on the leech to get these two initial folds right. Put a sail tie around them at the aft end.

Now work from slide to slide up the luff, pulling the luffrope between each slide to alternate sides to give the desired concertina effect. Return to the lowest slide and hold it while the person at the leech pulls back on the sail to create the folds.

The commonest mistake is to rush things, and not work as a pair. You must work on the same fold at the same time, or you will finish up with a dog's breakfast.

TIDYING UP THE BOAT

Clip the halyards to their stowages. On a cruising boat these should be somewhere other than on the mast, where they will clank remorsely all night long.

Coil the halyard, sheet and control line tails. There is a neat way to do this, using a winch. Stand facing the winch with the loose tail at your feet. Use your right hand to pass the line round and over the winch and back to your left hand to form a loop. Hold the end of the loop with your left hand and continue to loop over the winch and back, building up the coils evenly until the line is used up. Unless there are specific stowages you can leave the coiled lines hung on the winches.

Coil the mainsheet, passing the tail through the top of the coil to make a hanger which can then be hitched to the boom, thus keeping the mainsheet neatly coiled and off the deck. If it rains the mainsheet will not be lying in a sodden heap next time you come to use it.

Move the mainsheet traveller car out to one end of the traveller; this parks the boom off-centre and prevents those emerging from the main hatch braining themselves on it. Stowing the boom off-centre also keeps the cockpit clear. If the boat is lying alongside, move the boom to the outboard side.

9 Sail changing and reefing

If the wind gets up – or starts to die – the skipper will want to keep the boat sailing well by reducing or increasing sail. Depending on the boat, you do this by changing sails or altering their size – a process known as reefing.

CHANGING HEADSAILS

On a sailing yacht this is the equivalent of changing gear. The yacht may have two or three different-sized headsails used for different wind strengths. The biggest is used in the lightest breeze; as the breeze builds you will need to change to a smaller headsail. If it drops again you will need to change back.

Racing yachts have developed sail changing into a slick art: one sail goes up, the other comes down, and the yacht barely misses a step or drops more than one or two-tenths of a knot in speed. Such finesse requires not merely co-ordinated crew work and a lot of practice, but also a duplication of specialised gear which many cruising yachts do not carry.

When cruising we are less obsessed by speed and more concerned with safety and comfort. There are usually fewer people available to do the task, and those that are available will want to stay dry while doing it. If this means slower sail changes, fine.

On the other hand, the longer any job on board takes, the more opportunity there is for something to go wrong, so it often pays to be slick. This is particularly relevant when you are changing sails to suit a rising wind, since the longer you leave it the more difficult it becomes. A fast sail change in good time can save a lot of needless sweat and toil.

▽ When the sky darkens and the wind gets up it is time to reduce sail.

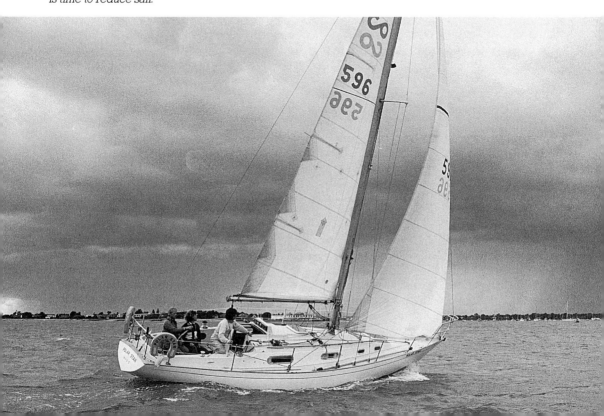

Bare-headed changing

The easiest way to change the headsail is to take down the old sail, take it off, put it away and then start again by bringing out the new sail, attaching it, hoisting it and sheeting in, leaving the yacht to sail along with no headsail (bare-headed) in the meantime.

There is nothing wrong with this method except that it takes time, and a yacht sailing under mainsail alone often has an awkward motion. Also, you must be careful to secure the halyard and sheets; if you leave them loose while you put the old sail away and drag out the new one, they will inevitably foul something while your back is turned.

A neater method is to get the new sail on deck, into the pulpit and hanked to the forestay (but still in its bag) before bringing the old sail down. Once the old sail is safely secured you can hoist the new sail, sheet it home and then clear up. This method reduces both the down-time when the yacht is not sailing efficiently and the time and effort needed to tend the sheets and halyard during the transfer. Here's how you do it.

1 With the new sail properly bagged so that the luff of the sail is at the mouth of the bag and the head, tack and clew are easily to hand, bring the bag into the pulpit and secure it.

2 If there are two tack eyes or shackles fitted to

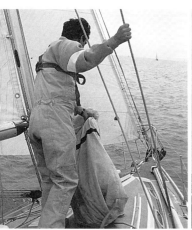

⌂ *Take the new sail forward.*

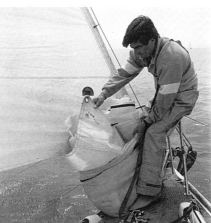

Find the tack, clew and head . . .

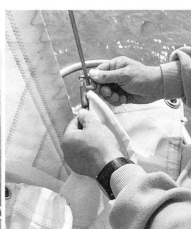

And hank it on.

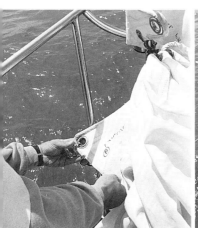

⌂ *Shackle the tack to the bow fitting . . .*

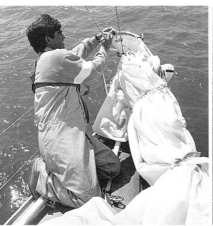

Shackle the halyard to the head of the new sail . . .

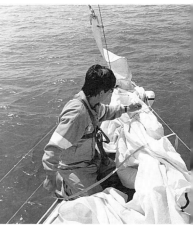

Undo any ties holding the sail to the rail . . .

the boat, attach the tack of the new sail on the spare one (if not, you will have to wait until the old sail is down before transferring the tack of the new sail to the tack shackle).

3 Hank the new sail onto the forestay, if necessary first dropping off one or two lower hanks of the old sail.

4 Drop the old sail. It is obviously quicker and handier if there are two of you, as one can tend the halyard or sheets while the other works the foredeck, but the job can easily be done by one. It just takes longer, and involves more running around.

5 With the old sail down, quickly detach the halyard and secure it to the pulpit or head of the new sail. Unhank the old sail from the forestay and put a sail tie around it, securing it to the pulpit and guardrail.

6 Release the sheets from the cockpit end and pull the clew of the old sail up to meet the head and tack in the pulpit. Detach the sheets and transfer them to the new sail; because the sail was packed properly (see Chapter 8) you will be able to do this with the sail still in its bag.

7 Reset the position of the sheet leads on their sliders; the sheeting position for the new sail will be different from that required for the old sail.

You now have the old sail in the bow, with the head, tack and clew all together along with

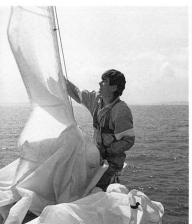
Drop the old sail . . .

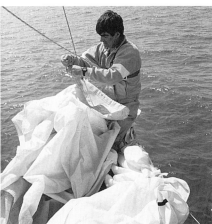
Unshackle the halyard, stow it, and . . .

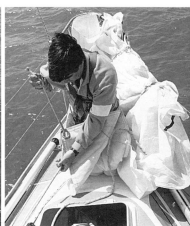
Tie the lee sheet to the new sail.

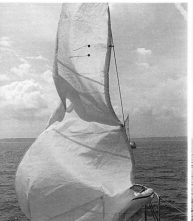
And haul on the halyard to raise it.

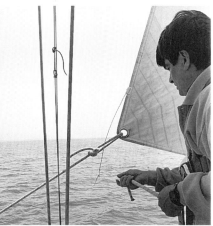
Tension the lee sheet to get the yacht sailing . . .

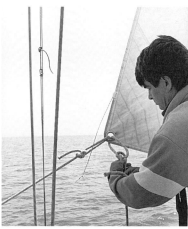
And attach the weather sheet.

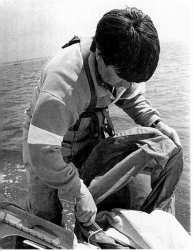
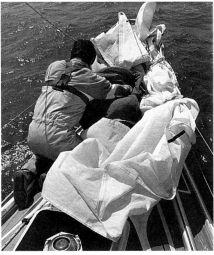
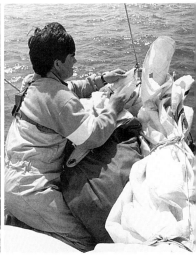

⌂ Bag the old sail from the leech end (nearest the mast).

Keep bundling it in the bag until you reach the forestay...

Then remove the hanks and tack to complete the job.

the luff, and the bunt of the sail doubled back along the foredeck; in other words, perfectly poised for bagging. Why not bag the old sail now, instead of hauling it aft in a great heap?

Start at the aft end of the doubled-over sail, and pull the bag up over everything until you reach the front. Release the sail ties securing the sail to the rail, unhook the tack, and you now have the sail bagged and ready for convenient re-use.

A racing crew would be appalled at the thought of bundling the sail, like so much straw,

into the bag. They are used to folding the sail on deck before bagging it. This is fine if you have a full crew, and necessary if you are sailing with sails made of stiff racing cloth. It is mandatory if you are using sails incorporating Kevlar, that brownish bulletproof material used in racing sails (Kevlar is so stiff you cannot just crunch it up even if the horrified owner would allow you to try). But cruising sails are normally (certainly should be) made of softer cloth, tighter woven but using less filler, and are more tolerant of such unceremonious treatment.

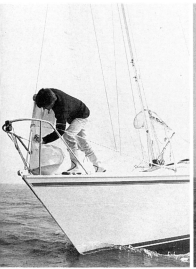
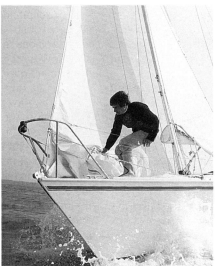
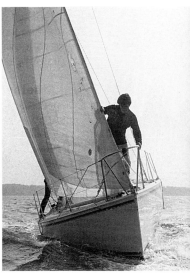

Variations

If the yacht has a grooved headstay, you must remember to use the pre-feeder (the D-shaped ring on the end of a wire strop connected to the tack fitting) before fitting the head of the sail into the groove.

You can of course do a bare-headed change, but if the boat has a twin luff-groove, the chances are that she is a yacht sometimes used for racing and has more than one headsail halyard (or one wire headsail halyard and two rope spinnaker halyards). This means you can go in for the sort of time-saving changes which are normal on racing yachts; the side-by-side method or the tack change.

Both these techniques are described, along with other racing tricks, in my book *Racing Crew*, so here only an outline is given.

In the side-by-side change you hoist the new sail on the spare halyard alongside the old sail. Depending on which groove and halyard the old sail is using, the new sail goes up either inside or outside the old sail. The important thing to remember is to use the halyard which is on the same side of the old sail as the new sail will be; otherwise the halyards will become crossed as the old sail comes down.

↶ *If the yacht has a twin-groove headfoil you can try a tack change, raising the new sail on the inside of the old one, tacking and dropping the old sail as the boat comes through the wind.*

The new sail is sheeted using either a spare sheet or a special changing sheet. If this is to work properly there have to be two sheet leads on each side of the boat. Alternatively you can feed the new sheet through the old lead position, and adjust it once the change is made. Once the new sail is sheeted in, bring down the old sail and take it off.

If the sail change has to be done while beating, a tack change is neater. Sail the boat on whichever tack puts the old sail in the outboard groove, and hoist the new sail inside the old sail. Lead the new sheet to the windward side and through a sheet lead adjusted to what will be the correct position for the new sail.

When the new sail is up and the halyard set, the yacht is tacked. Let go the old sheet and haul in the new sheet, attached to the new sail. Meanwhile the old halyard is let go as the yacht comes through the wind, allowing the old sail to come neatly down on deck.

REEFING

Reefing is reducing the size of a sail without actually taking it off, and is accomplished by folding up and securing the bottom part of the sail in a neat roll, and using only the upper part. Since most yachts carry only one mainsail, it is the normal method of reducing sail area aft of the mast – but many cruising yachts also carry reefing headsails.

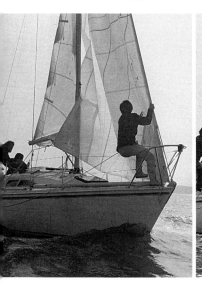
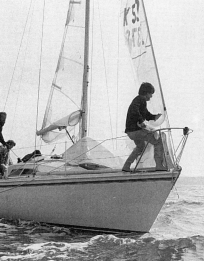
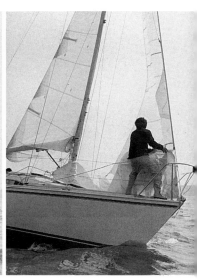

Reefing the headsail

The sail itself must be fitted for reefing, with a spare tack cringle in the luff above the normal tack cringle and a corresponding clew cringle for the sheets, some way up the leech above the normal clew. Both these cringles must have reinforcing patches around them, or the sail will quickly pull out of shape and become useless in its unreefed state.

To reef, start by easing the sheet to take the weight out of the sail; then ease the halyard until the new tack cringle meets the tack fitting on deck, and secure the tack. Transfer the sheet to the reefed clew position and reposition the sheet lead to suit the reefed sail; it will probably have to come forward. Retension the halyard and re-sheet the sail, making a final adjustment to the sheet lead if necessary.

You now have the sail set but with a large flap of cloth hanging loose underneath. Roll up the cloth and secure the roll with the attached cords, or reef pennants.

Curiously enough, you do not use reef knots for this. Instead, you tie a bow but pull one end right through. When you come to unreef you only have to pull the loose tail and the knot comes undone: much easier than breaking your

fingernails trying to undo a wet, tightened reef knot.

Roller furling headsails

All this seamanlike stuff is rendered redundant on a yacht with a roller furling headsail, where you change the headsail size merely by rolling up (or out) the desired amount of cloth.

The knack when shortening sail in this way is to keep the sheet under control while winding-in on the furlong line. If too much weight is in the sail, the rolls become too tight and all the line is wound in before the sail is fully furled. If the sheet and sail are simply let fly, you get a very untidy roll.

Roller-furling headsails are very convenient when sailing short-handed, but they rarely set well when part-furled. For this reason many skippers prefer to change sails, particularly if they can get someone else (such as you) to do the job for them.

Reefing the mainsail

Exactly the same principles apply as when reefing a headsail, except that the mainsail has the added complication of the boom. If you just drop the halyard, you will drop the boom onto

⇨ To reef the main, slacken the halyard and pull some sail down   *Slip the new tack cringle onto the reefing hook and retension the halyard.*   *The topping lift will hold the boom up.*

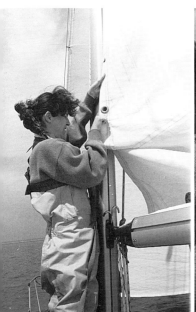
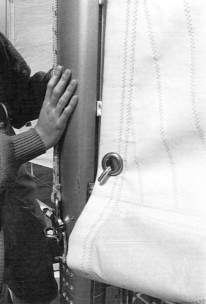
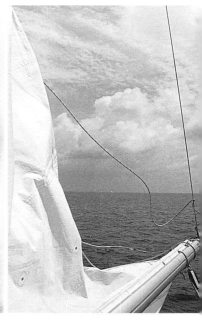

the coachroof and possibly onto someone's head. You need to support the boom by using the topping lift.

1 Ease the vang and the mainsheet.

2 Take the weight of the outboard end of the boom on the topping lift.

3 Ease the halyard so you can hook the reef cringle to the reefing hook, or to the gooseneck if you are using an inboard pennant.

4 Secure the cringle, then tension the halyard.

5 Tension the foot using the outboard end pennant, on a winch if necessary.

6 Ease off the topping lift and tension the mainsheet and vang.

7 The sail should now be able to set properly, ignoring the 'bunt', or bag of spare material; this is tidied up by tying off the reef pennants (between the sail and the boom if the sail has foot slides).

When reefing the mainsail the essential things to remember are:

• Take all the weight out of the sail, so you do not expend energy fighting against, say, the pull of the mainsheet.

• Retension the luff before you tension the foot.

• Make sure you finish with the sail held only by its three corners; there should be no weight on the eyelets in the sail which take the reef pennants or the continuous reefing line.

This last is very important. Weight on these eyelets will only pull the middle of the sail out of shape. They are there only to hold the rolled-up bunt of sail.

Roller reefing

You may come across a yacht with roller reefing, an older method of reefing the mainsail by rolling it around the boom like a roller blind. You wind the sail on to the boom using a crank fitted at the gooseneck, but otherwise the same principles apply. Take the weight of the boom on the topping lift and ease the mainsheet before starting.

Since the sail is wrapped around the boom, anything attached to the boom other than at the extreme ends must be taken off. This may include the mainsheet and certainly the vang, if there is one. Roller-reefed yachts often have the mainsheet fitted to the very end of the boom, or use a claw fitting for mainsheet, vang or both. If a claw is used, ensure that it does not poke into (or through) the fabric of the rolled sail. You may need to use padding.

Tension the reefing pennant to pull the new clew out and down.

Winch it tight to tension the foot of the sail . . .

And tie up the bunt of the sail through the eyelets.

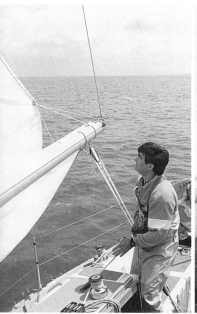
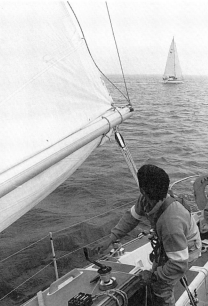
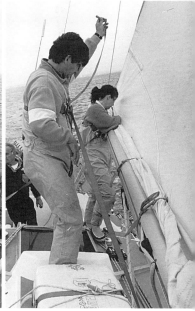

10 Spinnakers

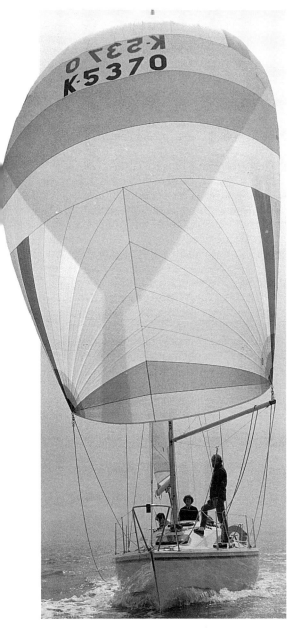

This yacht has double control lines. From left, they are: lazy (unused) guy, sheet, jibsheet over pole, guy and lazy sheet.

The sail area that is adequate and comfortable for a yacht sailing upwind is usually less than she needs going downwind. The reason is very simple: going into the wind, the speed of the yacht and the speed of the wind combine to give the speed, and thus the weight, of the wind across the sails. Going downwind, the speed of the yacht detracts from the speed of the wind, so although the true wind speed is the same, it *feels* as if there is less wind.

Being under-canvased is almost as uncomfortable for the yacht and her crew as being over-canvased; the yacht just slops along: it is sluggish to respond to the helm, the motion is jerky and unpredictable, things crash and bang around. Life is tedious. So to correct this malaise, extra sail is set.

The most usual sail is a large and lightweight sail called the spinnaker (it was first set on a yacht called *Sphinx*, and was so big it quickly became nicknamed 'sphinx's acre' – or so the story goes). Because of its size and relative complexity of handling, the spinnaker is often thought of as a racing sail. This is a great shame, because when used with common sense it can add enormously to the pleasure of cruising. It will keep the rate of progress up when the wind is light on a downwind course, and help to balance the yacht, making her easier to steer and live aboard, when the breeze is fresher.

Spinnakers *can* become difficult when used in marginal circumstances; the delight of cruising as opposed to racing is that when conditions are marginal you can leave the spinnaker in its bag. No less than five chapters of *Racing Crew* are devoted to spinnakers and the things that may be done with them. For the cruising crew the repertoire need not be so extensive, so only basic spinnaker handling is covered here.

How the spinnaker is rigged

The spinnaker is a big, symmetrical sail that is roughly hemispherical in shape when set. It flies above and before the yacht rather like a kite (indeed, it is often referred to as the 'kite').

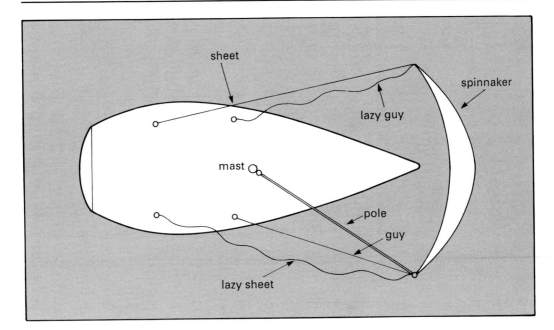

It is extended away from the boat on the windward side by the spinnaker pole and trimmed, like other sails, by a sheet.

The spinnaker has its own gear, consisting of halyard, pole, sheet and guy. The guy is the line that goes to the outboard end of the pole to hold it in place; the pole is supported by its own topping lift and held down by the downhaul or foreguy.

When set, the spinnaker flies outside the forestay, and the headsail is usually taken down so as not to interfere with the flow of air into the spinnaker.

HOISTING THE SPINNAKER

One competent person can set and handle a spinnaker under cruising conditions, but life is easier with two or, better still, three. This allows one to do the foredeck work, including helping with the halyard, and two to share the halyard work and look after the sheet and guy. With fewer people, you just have to run around a bit more. The secret of success is to get everything prepared beforehand.

To set the spinnaker you need:
● The sail on deck, in the pulpit, but still in its bag (which is secured to something to stop it blowing overboard).

● The sheet and guy led outside everything to the correct corners of the sail, and clipped on.
● The halyard attached to the head of the sail.
● The guy led through the outboard end of the pole.
● The pole attached to the mast and supported horizontally by the topping lift.
● The sheet and guy led to their respective winches in the cockpit.

When ready to hoist, you need:
● Someone on the halyard.
● Someone on the sheet.
● Someone on the guy.

The difficult time is the period between the sail being safely in its bag and the sail being safely aloft, set and drawing; keep this time as short as possible.

Start by 'cheating the guy': pulling the guy aft so that the clew of the sail comes out of the bag and up to the pole.

Next, heave quickly and firmly on the halyard to hoist the sail to the masthead. As the sail reaches the top, bring the guy and pole aft to help the sail open and fill.

When the sail is up and the guy aft – and not before – haul the sheet in and the spinnaker will blossom. when you are satisfied all is well, lower the headsail to the deck and either secure it to the guardrail or take it off completely.

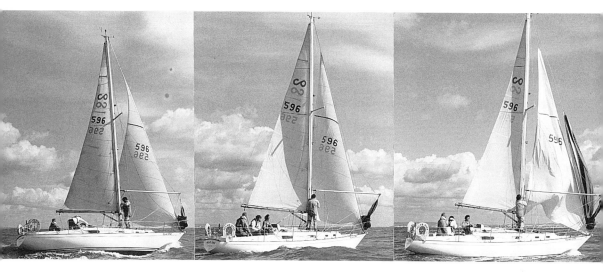

⌂ *With the sail still in its bag, attach the sheet and guy and rig the pole.*

Pull the guy aft to drag the clew of the sail out of the bag and up to the pole . . .

Then take the halyard and heave the sail to the masthead.

Common faults

- *Taking too long.* The half-up, half-filled spinnaker flicks and flogs around all over the place, eventually wrapping itself around anything it can find. Delay in hoisting is usually the result of not having everything ready beforehand.
- *Leaving it too long to bring the guy aft.* With the pole still on the forestay, the spinnaker is blanketed by the headsail and will not fill.
- *Hauling the sheet in too soon.* The sail will be pulled into the back of the headsail and the shadow of the mainsail, and will not fill; or, if the guy has also been brought aft too quickly, the sail will fill before the halyard is up and secured. When this happens, it is at best hard work with a winch to get the sail properly hoisted; at worst the halyard is ripped out of your hands, the sail goes in the water ahead of the boat and the boat sails over the spinnaker (not good news). Fortunately, releasing the sheet again can usually solve most problems before they develop.
- *Leaving the sheet too late.* The head of the sail spins a couple of times as it is pulled aloft, putting a twist in the sail which, when the sheet is pulled, fills in the classic 'wineglass' twist with the top and bottom swelling nicely but apparently joined together by a tight nylon knot.

Undoing a twist

Let go the sheet and at the same time ease the pole forward, then grab the luff of the sail and pull downwards while easing the halyard two or three feet.

If the twist does not come out with a couple of quick tugs, admit defeat and pull the whole sail down onto the foredeck. Find the luff tape at the pole end and run it through your fingers back up towards the head, pulling off the twist when you reach it. Holding that luff tape, hoist the sail again, letting the tape run through your fingers.

TRIMMING THE SPINNAKER

The golden rules are:
- The spinnaker should be symmetrical about its vertical midline.
- The pole should be at right angles to the direction of the wind, as shown by the masthead burgee or wind indicator.
- The two corners of the sail, the tack and clew, should be level. Since the clew (the corner with the sheet attached) finds its own level, the outboard end of the pole with the tack attached needs to be adjusted to suit the clew. Doing it the other way round does not work.

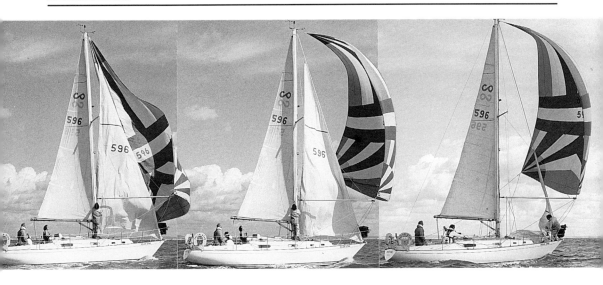

As the sail starts to fill, pull on the guy to bring the pole aft . . .

Then sheet in. The spinnaker should blossom.

If all is well, lower the headsail and either secure it or stow it.

↶ *A classic 'wineglass' spinnaker twist.*

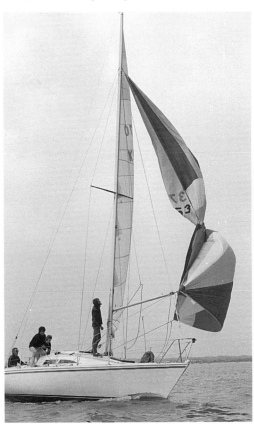

• The pole itself should be horizontal, so once the sail is set and the outboard end of the pole has been adjusted, level the pole by raising or lowering the inboard end.

When you are controlling the sheet, the rule is the same as with any other sail: let it out until it flaps, then pull it in. As you ease the sheet, you will see the luff of the spinnaker start to curl as the sail begins to backwind. Stop easing the sheet and bring it in until the curl just disappears.

Common faults

• *Pole too for forward.* The sail keeps collapsing, but from the top or even the middle rather than from the luff, as it would if the sheet was eased too much. Because the pole is too far forward the sail itself has to be pulled too far round and gets under the shadow of the mainsail, so the flow of air into the sail is unstable and unpredictable.

• *Pole too far aft.* The sail collapses from the luff, and it can be made to set only if the sheet is pulled so tight that the foot of the sail stretches taut across the forestay.

• *Pole outboard end too low.* The corners are not level, with the clew and its sheet floating higher than the tack at the pole end. The windward luff of the sail is too tight.

• *Pole outboard end too high.* The corners are

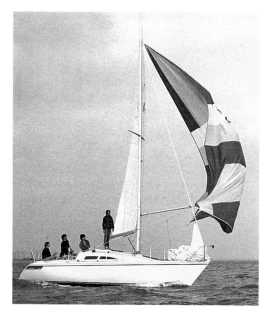

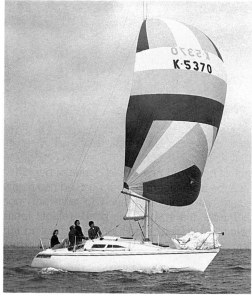

not level, but the clew with its sheet hangs down below the level of the tack and the pole; the windward luff of the sail is too loose and bellies upwards, twisting the whole sail. The pole height is right when both edges of the sail follow matching curves.

• *Sheet too tight (over-sheeting)*. The foot of the sail becomes taut or even straight, choking the bottom of the sail. The flow of air over the spinnaker is quite complex: air enters from both sides, meets in the middle and mostly flows downwards off the sail, so it is important to keep the bottom of the sail open to let the air off and thus allow more air on.

Rolling

If the spinnaker is carried too high as the breeze increases it can set up an unpleasant and eventually dangerous rolling motion which gets worse as the sail starts to sway in harmony with the roll. This can be cured quite easily by taking the lead of the sheet forward, even as far forward as the shrouds, to pull the clew down and flatten the spinnaker, and then lowering the tack (and pole) to match.

GYBING THE SPINNAKER

This is essentially a matter of shifting the spinnaker pole from one side of the sail to the other,

▵ With the pole too far forward (left) the luff and leech fall together; if it is too far back (right) the luff falls in and the foot is tight across the forestay.

so the original guy becomes the new sheet, and vice versa. There are two methods of doing this; the one you use is dictated largely by the type of pole the yacht carries.

End-for-end

If the boat has a double-ended pole you can use the end-for-end method.

With the boat running square off the wind, unship the inboard end of the pole from the mast. Release the old guy from the outboard end by tripping the end plunger, leaving the pole hanging on the topping lift bridle. Drop what will be the new guy into what was the inboard end and move the pole across the boat, pushing out the new guy, until you can clip the new inboard end on to the mast fitting.

Dip pole

If the yacht has a single-ended pole the inboard end stays on the mast while you swing the pole across the boat, lowering (dipping) the outboard end to allow it to pass under the forestay.

For this method, the spinnaker has to be equipped with double lines (a separate sheet and guy) to each corner of the sail.

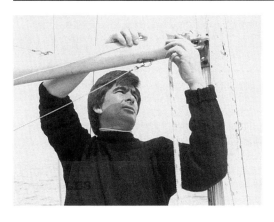
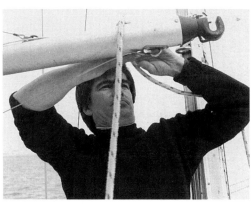

⌂ End-for-end gybe. (1) Stand at the mast facing forward and unclip the pole.

⌂ (2) Drop the new headsail sheet over the end and pass the pole across the boat.

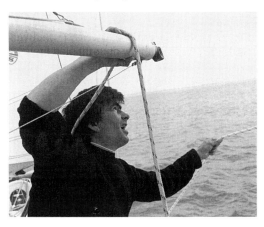
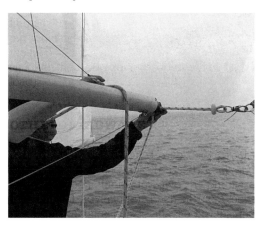

⌂ (3) Grab the new guy, and . . .

⌂ (4) Fit the guy into the pole end.

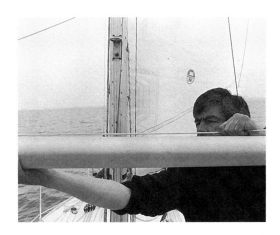
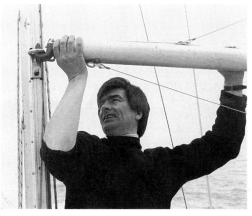

⌂ (5) Trip the other end and drop the old headsail sheet off.

⌂ (6) Clip on.

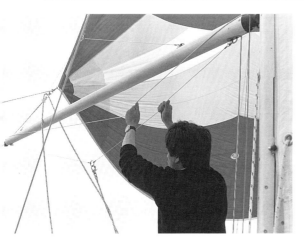

⟲ *A dip-pole gybe. (1) Trip the pole end.*

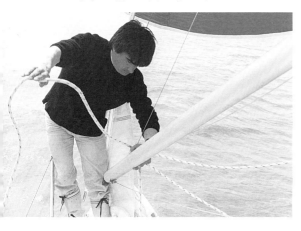

⟲ *Dip the pole and swing it across.*
⟲ *Clip the pole to the new guy, raise it and winch it aft before trimming the sheet.*

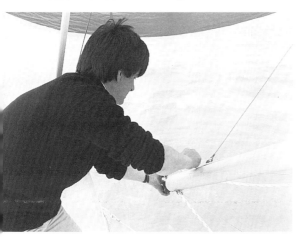

Sheet and guy during the gybe

These have to be tended so that the sail floats high and wide, without collapsing, throughout the gybe. As the outboard end of the pole comes off, the old guy will need to be eased a little, then brought in to keep the sail full as the boat turns in the gybe.

The old sheet (new guy) must be eased to allow the pole to be set on the new side.

Mainsail and helm during the gybe

It greatly helps if the mainsail is kept close to the centreline while the spinnaker is gybed, for this will help keep the spinnaker full. If the spinnaker is gybed before the mainsail, it will not fill on the new side. It will collapse and stands a good chance of wrapping itself round the forestay.

If the mainsail is gybed fully before the pole is shifted across (common practice in dinghies) the spinnaker will probably collapse either because there is nothing to support what has now become the guy and windward side of the sail, or because the sail is blanketed by the main.

The golden rule for the helmsman is 'Keep The Boat Under The Spinnaker'. Turning too fast or too far, or not turning enough, will put the spinnaker out to one side or the other and trigger a chain reaction of imbalance which will probably result in a collapse, a wrap, a broach, or all three.

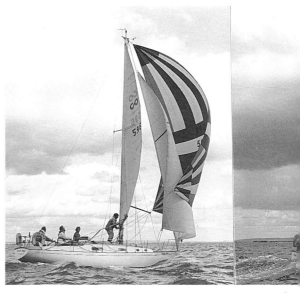

Just how far to turn depends on the weight of wind. Basically, the more wind there is, the narrower the turn, not least because the need to keep the mainsail sheeted close until the spinnaker is gybed calls for the yacht to be sailed dead downwind.

If you think there is too much wind to gybe safely with the spinnaker up, take the sail off, gybe, and re-set it.

LOWERING THE SPINNAKER

The expression 'dropping the spinnaker' often too accurately describes what takes place; the aim is not to drop it, but to lower it. There are various sophisticated techniques employed in racing, but only one, the safest and easiest, is described here.

You want to take the spinnaker down in the lee of the other sails, where the wind in it will cause no problems. This is easiest going almost dead downwind; the more of a reach the yacht is on, the less easy it is to kill the spinnaker behind the main before taking it down.

First, set the headsail. Then ease the guy and the pole forward to the forestay, taking up on the foreguy to keep the pole under control. This in itself will partly collapse the sail.

Grab the sheet (or lazy guy if fitted) and take this up the lee side, under the boom, to amidships.

Let the guy run through the pole end, and at the same time gather in the foot of the sail along its foot-tape, behind the mainsail. You should now have a long nylon sausage hanging from the mast behind the mainsail. Let the halyard off and keep it under control as you bring the sail down and gather it under the boom, passing it down below as you do so.

Common faults

• *Letting the sail go in the water.* This is usually caused by letting off the halyard too soon or too quickly, but it may also result from trying to gather the sail too close to the rail, and dropping some of it over the side.

• *Sailing too high.* You need to sail directly downwind while the spinnaker comes off. The more you sail across the wind the more pressure there is in the sail, the more the yacht is heeled and the more difficult it all becomes. Something will go wrong, and you risk losing a crew member over the side.

• *Leaving it all too late.* The more wind, the more difficulty. As the breeze rises and the yacht surfs gloriously along, it is easy to forget that eventually the spinnaker is going to have to come off. When that time comes, you're in trouble.

▷ *To lower the spinnaker first set the headsail, ease the guy and sheet forward, haul in on the sheet and bring the sail down.*

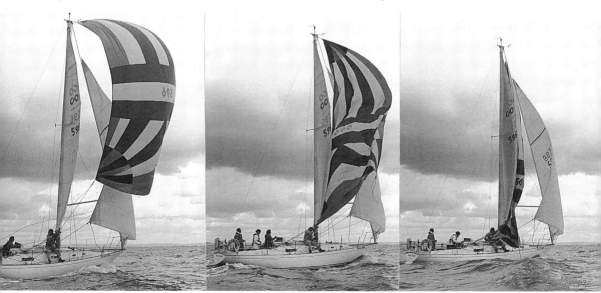

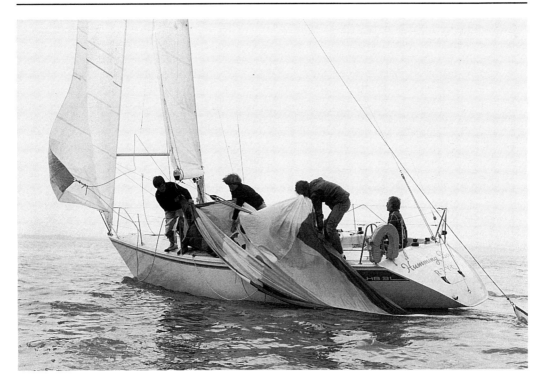

⌂ *If the spinnaker goes overboard retrieve it by pulling one tape at a time to spill the water from the sail.*

SPINNAKER SOCKS

Spinnaker socks can take a lot of the grief out of spinnaker handling. The sock is a long cylinder of (usually) nylon cloth, in which the spinnaker is stowed. At its lower end is a bell-shaped mouth of glassfibre or stiffened fabric, and at its upper end is a block with a continuous light line passing through it. The line is long enough to lead all the way from the bottom of the sock to the top and back again, with some to spare.

You hoist the spinnaker inside its sock, with the sheet and guy made up in the normal way, and the pole rigged. With the tack at the pole end under tension, you use the light line to pull the bell-mouth up towards the head of the sail, pulling the sock up with it, while tensioning the sheet. This releases the spinnaker and allows it to fill from the bottom.

The bell-mouth and folded-up sock remain at the head of the spinnaker all the time the sail is set.

To lower or even gybe the sail, the spinnaker is first smothered by releasing the sheet (thus dumping the wind from the sail) and hauling down on the line from the bell-mouth.

Advantages
The most troublesome part of spinnaker handling, the setting and lowering of the sail, is greatly simplified.

Disadvantages
The sock and its bell-mouth have to stay on top of the spinnaker all the time it is up. This marginally detracts from performance, but more seriously it can cause problems with chafe. All that crumpled cloth can also get trapped in the halyard and its fittings, or in something else aloft.

If the bell-mouth is on the small side, it can be a real problem hauling it down over the deflated spinnaker. You may need to take the downhaul line onto a winch, with consequent risk of damage to the sock or spinnaker. This problem is easily remedied by fitting a larger bell-mouth, but if you're new on board it might be more tactful to keep such suggestions to yourself for a bit.

11 Arriving

The way a yacht comes into a berth tells you a great deal about her crew. Poor teamwork at this stage is embarrassing and frustrating, and can be expensive or even dangerous if you miss your mooring and hit another boat.

The first priority is to have the yacht under full control. Arriving alongside under sail can be done (has to be done if the yacht has no engine, or the engine has broken down) but generally harbour masters and marina masters will become quite irritated if you arrive at the dock with the sails still up. So it is common practice to take the sails off (see Chapter 6) before you enter the marina, and come in under engine.

Lines and fenders
These should be brought out from their stowage in plenty of time, and rigged well before you arrive alongside.

⟁ Rig the fenders in good time, but stow them on deck until the final approach.

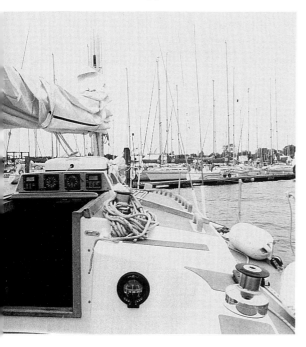

As far as lines go, you will need at least a head rope and stern rope. Make sure you select good, long lines; the head rope and stern rope should be at least as long as the yacht herself. Coil each neatly, but do not attach the end which stays on the boat (the bitter end) to its cleat just yet.

Get the fenders ready; two can be hung amidships, at the point where the yacht is widest (the point where the yacht's sides will rest against the berth) and at least one other should be kept in hand, to be placed where needed as the skipper makes the final approach to the berth. Fenders placed near the bow and stern will protect the yacht if she swings.

Some skippers will allow you to hitch the fender's line to the top guardrail, but others will have apoplexy if you try; the weight of the fender will cause the guardrail to sag and stretch, which some people hate. On the whole, it is more prudent to hitch fenders to the toerail, the stanchion bases and the handrail on the cabin top.

A neat method is to hitch the fender tail to the top guardrail, but at a stanchion, using a clove hitch with its two loops passed over the rail either side the stanchion head. This does not stretch the guardrail wire and does not leave the fender tail stretched across the side deck (the main problem with hitching it to the handrail on the cabin top). It is also convenient to get at if it needs to be adjusted.

Set the length of the fender tail so that the bottom of the fender is just kissing the water. It is rather neat to set the fenders properly, then bring them inboard again until the final approach to the berth, rather than have the yacht drive around with the fenders hanging over the side like a holiday hire boat crewed by trippers.

Standing around – McKeag's Law
As the yacht approaches the berth, everyone stands either where they are going to be needed once alongside, or where they will have

a good view of the impending crash. In either case the helmsman's view becomes increasingly obscured by legs, bottoms and backs at the moment when he most needs to see where he is going. So universal is this phenomenon that it can be mathematically stated as McKeag's Law; the number of people standing between a helmsman and an obstruction increases as the distance between the yacht and the obstruction decreases.

Do not fall victim to McKeag's Law. The best place to stand, or ideally sit, is along the centre-line of the boat, at the boom or the mast, leaving the helmsman with a clear view ahead and along either side deck.

Escape plan

Engines stop unexpectedly only when you need them; the steering gear fails only when you want to turn the yacht; the gear lever comes off in your hand only when you urgently need to shift gear. In view of this, the well-prepared yacht always has an escape plan formulated in case things go wrong.

This might involve anything from simply overshooting the berth and going round again, to quickly hoisting a sail or letting go the anchor, depending on circumstance. Preparing and initiating the escape plan is down to the skipper, but you the crew will have to put it into effect. If you have not been told what it is, or if there does not appear to be one – ask. Use tact. Asking 'What are we going to do when this goes wrong?' is unlikely to elicit a courteous response, but 'Do you want the mainsail cover

▷ *Always coil a spirally laid rope with the lay, or it will fall in a tangle (right).*

on now or shall we leave it off until we get alongside?' might well earn you a measure of (probably unspoken) gratitude.

Throwing a line

Nothing marks out a seaman (of either sex) more clearly than the way he or she can heave a line; nothing is more embarrassing than to stand there, coils in hand, with all eyes upon you, then have the whole lot flop feebly into the water in a tangle while the wind blows the yacht inexorably away from her berth. To avoid this indignity, learn to do it properly.

Coil the line carefully, using comfortable-sized coils; do not coil the line to the full stretch of your arms.

Wrap the bitter end (the end you want to retain) around your non-throwing hand, clamping the end under your thumb. Divide the coiled line between your two hands, holding rather less in your throwing hand than in the other.

Make sure you stand where the line, as you swing and throw it, will not catch on anything – the shrouds, for example – and where the momentum of your throw will not cause you to overbalance and topple overboard.

Swing your throwing arm back, forwards and back again, then carry through the return swing into the throw, heaving the line high and clear. Allow the coils in your other hand to run free, letting them fall off your hand as they are needed. The less drag the rest of the line inflicts on the coils you have thrown, the longer and cleaner will be the throw.

Do not throw the line directly at the person you think might catch it; throw the line above and beyond him, so that it falls across or beside him and is easy to pick up.

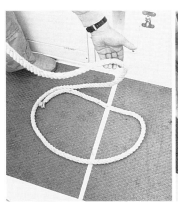
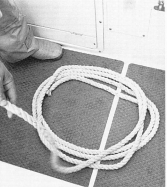
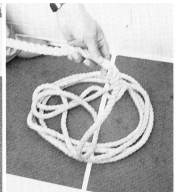

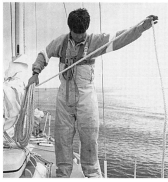
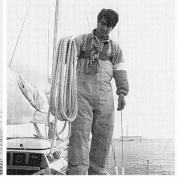
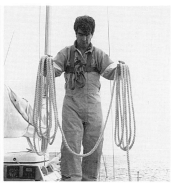

⌂ Coil the heaving line.　　　　Clamp one end with your thumb . . . And split the coil into two.

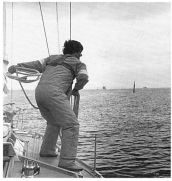
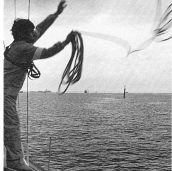
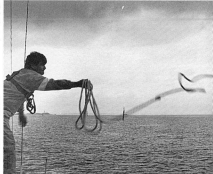

⌂ Select a good vantage point and swing one coil back . . .　　Heave the line high and clear so it unrolls in the air . . .　　And allow the coils to run free as needed.

Similarly, if you are trying to catch a line, do not worry about catching the end or even the line in your hand. Let it drop across your arm (a bigger, easier target) or fall beside you where you can stamp your foot on it to stop it running back off the dock into the water.

Hopping ashore

If there is no one on the dock to receive the lines, a crewmember must hop ashore to take them. The obvious place to stand would appear to be the bow, but remember that the intention is to arrive alongside – not bows-on or at an angle. As the yacht nears the pontoon the skipper will turn her alongside, and the bow will suddenly swing away, opening the distance between you and the dock just as you are about to jump. Most unfair.

The better place to stand ready to jump is at the shrouds, with both feet on the toerail outboard of the guardrails. That way you should be able to get ashore with one small step for a man, rather than one giant leap for mankind.

Stopping

Once the line is passed, get it around something quickly while you still have the chance. Remember that at the other end of the line is several tons of yacht still moving forward, eager to drag you off your feet. The image of the horror-struck crewman, leaning back on the line at 45 degrees and still moving at speed up the dock, smoke pouring from the soles of his boots, is too close to reality to be funny – especially if you are either the unfortunate crewman or the owner of the boat.

In contrast, there is *enormous* satisfaction to be gained from bringing several tons of yacht to a gentle halt simply by leaning your own puny weight against the pull of a rope you have nonchalantly dropped over the end of a cleat or round a mooring bollard.

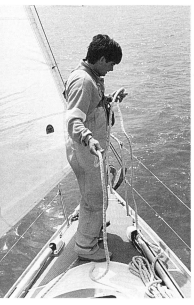 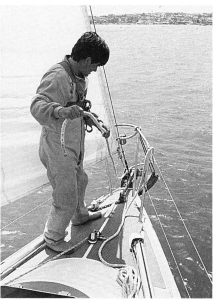 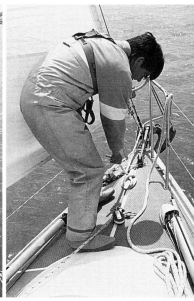

⌂ *Pass the end of a mooring line over the rail...*　　*Back through the fairlead on the toerail...*　　*And cleat it. This ensures that it runs fairly.*

On board, the same rule applies. As soon as the line is thrown and collected, pass the bitter end under the guardrail from the outside, through a fairlead and onto a cleat or winch. If the line is already secured to a cleat as you approach the dock, uncleat it and pass the end down *outside* the guardrail, through a fairlead and back onto the cleat before coiling the rest. This ensures that it falls fairly.

MOORING

The precise disposition of the mooring lines is the skipper's responsibility. The head rope and stern rope should be led well forward and aft, rather than brought straight ashore at right angles to the boat. Ideally you should lead the lines to cleats on the dock about half the boat's length ahead and astern of where she is lying, but you will probably have to make the most of what is available.

It is the springs which keep the boat in position; these are lines which run ashore aft from the bow and forward from the stern, crossing somewhere amidships. Again, the precise lead will depend on the securing points ashore. The most satisfactory arrangement is for the fore

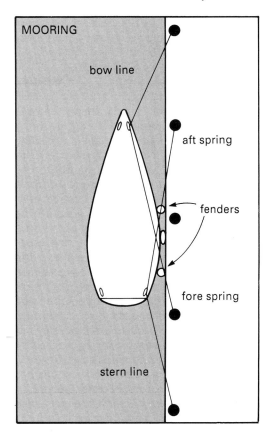

MOORING

bow line

aft spring

fenders

fore spring

stern line

spring to go from a cleat on board near (but not at) the bow to a bollard or cleat ashore level with the stern; and for the aft spring to go from a cleat on board near the stern to a point ashore level with the bow.

A less satisfactory but commonly-seen arrangement (thanks to the disposition of cleats on the average marina pontoon) is for both springs to be led ashore to a common cleat amidships.

The least satisfactory arrangement is for the long spare end of the head rope to be led back on board from its position ashore and secured on board somewhere towards the back of the boat, and the arrangement repeated but reversed for the long spare end of the stern rope. Although attractively economical with the use of mooring lines, this gives the springs too acute a lead for them to do their job properly, which is to check the boat's tendency to surge back and forth in her berth by pulling her against the dockside.

Mooring stern-on

If you are invited on a Mediterranean cruise you will almost certainly get involved in mooring stern-on to the dock. This is standard procedure in Mediterranean marinas, since it allows many more boats to be packed into the space available – but it can be a headache for the crew.

The basic idea is to moor the stern to the dock, and secure the bow to a mooring buoy or anchor. Here's how it's done.

If there are no mooring buoys, you drop the anchor some six to seven boat lengths from the wall and turn the boat around to aim the stern at your mooring slot. Go astern and slowly motor back towards the wall, paying out the anchor chain as necessary. If a mooring buoy is provided you will need to pick it up (see below) and pass the yacht's head rope through the ring. Secure it with a round turn and two half-hitches. You might prefer to bring it back aboard, rather than tying direct to the buoy. That way, when you come to leave you can simply slip the bow mooring – pull it through the ring – without having to undo a knot which, invariably, will have pulled tight. The problem with this is that the rope tends to chafe, so it is not recommended if you are mooring for more than an hour or so.

Secure two mooring lines to the cleats on the stern, one on each side, and pass them under the guardrails and through the fairleads. Take them ashore and cross them, so that the line from the starboard side goes to the port mooring bollard and the line from the port side goes to the starboard bollard. These will act as springs. Then pull forward on the anchor or the mooring buoy to heave the yacht some three feet off the dock. When you come to disembark you can haul on the mooring line to reduce the gap, and the yacht will spring back when you let go. Arriving back from ashore, you just pull the yacht in to the dock with the stern rope.

Be sure to use plenty of fenders on either side of the boat, since this system – and those whom you will meet using it – relies on the sardine effect to keep all the boats in place.

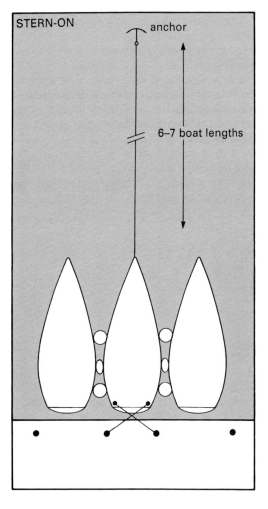

STERN-ON
anchor
6–7 boat lengths

PICKING UP A MOORING

Although marina-hopping is what passes for cruising for so many yachts, there is a special attraction in lying off. This means either anchoring or picking up a mooring.

Which mooring to pick up will again be a skipper's decision: it is a foolhardy skipper who simply picks up what looks like a free mooring without checking first that it really is free and that is really is a mooring, and not just a buoy marking the upper end of a piece of old, rotten chain.

Once he has decided, it will be the crew's job to secure the yacht to the buoy, while the master has the easy job of steering. The mooring will usually have some sort of pick-up buoy attached to a length of light line, to which is attached the real mooring rope, chain or wire.

On a small boat you can lie flat on the deck, with your head and one shoulder protruding through the feet of the pulpit, and pick up the buoy by hand.

A less heroic method is to use a boat-hook, but rather than attempt to spear its end through the ring or hand-loop on the top of the buoy (you will probably miss) it is better to go for the rope under the buoy.

As the buoy comes within reach, hold the boat-hook so that the hook itself is facing forward and sweep it underneath the buoy so that the staff of the boat-hook hits the vertical rope. No great accuracy is needed.

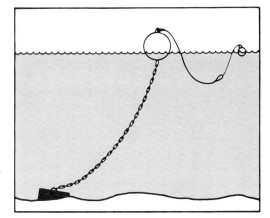

◇ A typical mooring. Note the way the pick-up buoy is attached to the real mooring rope.

Swiftly pull the boat-hook towards you; the rope will run along the staff until it is caught by the hook. As you lift the boat-hook clear of the water the pick-up buoy will flop over the other side of the hook, preventing the line from dropping off.

Reach through the front legs of the pulpit to grab the pick-up line, and use it to bring the mooring line on board. Normally, the pick-up line will be attached to a large loop in the mooring, and this loop is led through the bow fairlead and dropped over the mooring cleat.

Do make sure you have brought the real mooring aboard, and are not trying to secure the yacht with the pick-up line.

◇ With the boat-hook ready guide the boat to the mooring.

Sweep the boat-hook under the pick-up buoy to hook the line . . .

Haul in the mooring strop and drop it over the cleat.

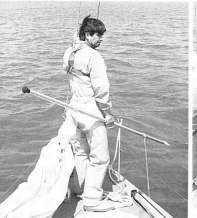

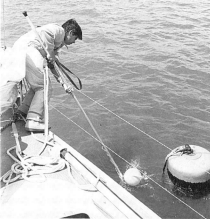

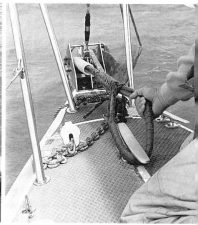

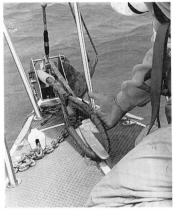 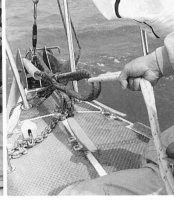 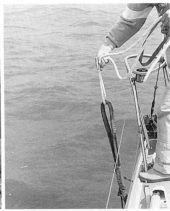

⌒ *If you try to slip the mooring strop like this you could trap your hand.*

Pass a loop of line through and use it to pull the strop off the cleat . . .

Then pass it amidships to allow the boat to bear off without fouling the line.

ANCHORING

Your cruising life will be the poorer if you never use it to find a spot away from all the others, away from marinas and crowded moorings. The anchor gives you the freedom to stop more or less where you will.

From a crewing point of view anchor work is relatively straightforward, since the skipper has to make the decisions about where to anchor, and when.

It is important to realise that it is not the anchor which holds the yacht, but the cable. The anchor holds the bottom end of the cable in place on the seabed, but the weight of the cable does the real work. For this reason the most satisfactory anchor cable is one composed entirely of chain, although for reasons of economy, weight-saving or supposed convenience many yachts are equipped with a short length of chain at the anchor end, the rest of the cable being rope.

An anchor with a rope cable and no chain at all is hardly worthy of the name, being properly called a kedge; it is used only for temporary anchoring and should never be thought of as secure. A popular name for such an arrangement is the 'lunch-hook', which tells the whole story.

⌒ *It is the long cable that anchors the boat; the anchor itself just holds the cable.*

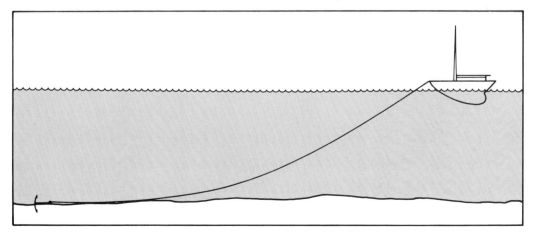

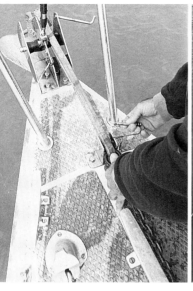

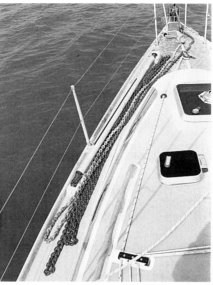

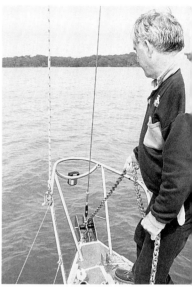

◠ *Remove the pins or lashings that secure the anchor.*

Flake the cable, securing the boat end on a cleat . . .

And lower the anchor over the bow ready to let go.

Making ready

On a large boat with a heavy anchor, there will probably be an anchor windlass with a 'gypsy': a toothed wheel over which the chain cable runs. The anchor is let go direct from its stowage position after being first 'cleared away'.

Take off the security lashings and remove the stowage pin, checking first that the brake on the gypsy is firmly on and that the chain is properly in the gypsy.

Using the brake on the gypsy (or by using power, if the yacht is big enough to have a

◡ *Raising the anchor may be a two-man job.*

Signal to the skipper when the anchor is clear of the water . . .

Then stow it, wash it off and stow the chain.

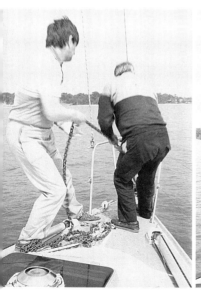

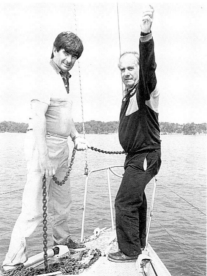

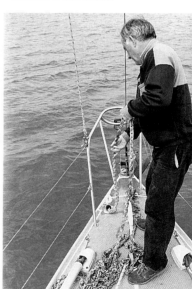

powered windlass), gently lower the anchor part-way clear of its stowage housing. You may have to use your hands or feet to start it moving – but be sure you can get your fingers or feet clear if it goes with a rush.

You want to have the anchor in such a position that it is clear to run without hanging-up on something once the order is given to let go, but you do not want it dangling in such a way that it swings against the hull with every swell.

On a smaller boat with no windlass the anchor is let go by hand, and the main priority is to make sure that the cable is free to run. From the chain hole in the deck (from now on call it the navel pipe) or the anchor well, pull up as much cable as the skipper says you will need, and flake it (lay it in long loops side by side, rather than coils) back along the foredeck, maybe as far back as the shrouds.

Bring the anchor itself out through the pulpit legs at the bow and lift it over the rail and onto the deck.

When the time comes to let go, do not fling the anchor away from the boat with a mighty heave: at best you will get wet from the splash, but at worst you will pull a muscle or even find you are standing with one foot inside a loop of the now fast-running cable.

Instead, lower the anchor slowly over the bow by the cable, then take the weight of the cable and anchor inboard of the pulpit; when the moment comes, simply let go, making sure you are not standing on the flaked cable or inside one of its loops.

Before giving the order to let go, the skipper (if coming to anchor under sail) should have turned the boat head to wind or current (which-ever is stronger) and waited for her to stop and begin to drift backwards; if manoeuvring under power a well-timed kick astern has the yacht moving gently backwards as the anchor is let go. In this way the cable does not fall in a heap on top of the anchor, but is laid out neatly on the seabed behind it, ready to take the weight of the boat.

When the yacht takes her anchor, she will turn with her head towards it and the cable. You can watch for this satisfying moment by looking at the land over the stern. Suddenly, the stern will start to swing quite fast; that is the yacht feeling and turning to her anchor. You have arrived.

12 Emergencies

When you go on your first trip with an experienced crew it's easy to assume that they have all the answers, and that nothing will go dramatically wrong. Unfortunately you have no guarantee of this, and if there is an emergency you may find that you are the only person in a fit state to deal with it. You need to know how.

MAN OVERBOARD

Falling overboard has been called the ultimate horror. The only question is who is the more horrified – the person in the water or the people left on board who have to get him back? Either way their horror is justified, for this is an accident that can easily turn into a tragedy.

The best solution is to avoid the problem altogether. When there is the slightest risk, you must wear safety harnesses. Some advocate that children should wear safety harnesses all

the time: but if the kids need them, how much more do Mum and Dad need them, for what can the kids do if Mum or Dad slips and goes over? Safety harnesses are not simply for the young or inexperienced: the senior members of the crew, including the skipper, should wear theirs also, if only for the peace of mind of the others.

Much the same applies to personal buoyancy. A full lifejacket is a cumbersome thing to wear all the time, and certainly this book does not advocate so doing, for anyone other than small children – but a jacket with personal buoyancy is so sensible a precaution that not to wear one on all but the quietest days seems foolhardy. Choose a jacket that has a security strap which fits under your crotch, to stop the jacket floating off over your head just when you need it most. The best jackets have a safety-harness built-in, and need only the addition of the tether-line.

◁ Safety harnesses and lifejackets are essential for small children – even in port.

◁ If your jacket has a built-in safety harness you are more likely to use it.

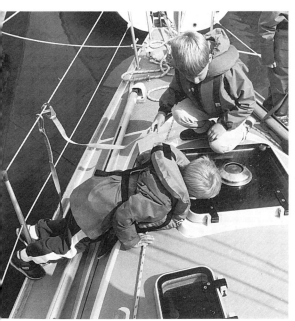

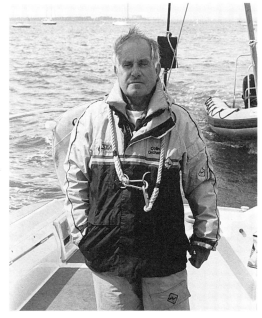

Recovery: practice beforehand

Retrieving the situation has three distinct phases, each with its own problems which you should think out in advance – both personally, and as a matter of the yacht's routine: getting back to the person in the water; getting that person back on board; and keeping that person alive once they are back on board.

One way to take some of the terror out of the situation is to practise beforehand. Many crews practise 'man-overboard drill': they throw over a fender, then have everyone take turns at bringing the yacht back alongside. It is worth doing both under sail and under engine, and is often rather fun, as well as being useful, not to say essential, practice. Even if you never have to do it for real (and God forbid that you do) it is a great way for every member of the crew to become familiar with handling the boat, and a great way to develop everyone's confidence.

But who then ever goes on to practise getting the person back on board? In truth, in the real situation this is going to be at least as difficult, if not far more so, than simply getting the boat back to the person in the water. In all but warm seas (the Mediterranean in summer, or the Caribbean) an individual in the sea has

⟡ Make sure you know where the lifebelts are, just in case . . .

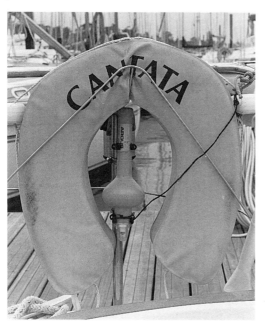

between five minutes and half-an-hour before cold begins seriously to sap his or her strength. With a high-sided yacht it is impossible for a fully-conscious, fully-fit person to do it unaided, so a chilled, exhausted, waterlogged man, woman or child has no chance.

One way to get even half a handle on the problem is to take a suit of oilskins of the jacket-and-high-trousers variety. Tie off the ankles and wrists and make up a dummy by stuffing the suit with some old sweaters, a sleeping bag or whatever. Put the trousers over the jacket, with the braces crossed over where the head would be, and put the whole thing in a lifejacket, tying the sleeves across and then tying it all together with light line. Use this instead of the fender – and (providing the whole lot does not disintegrate on you the first time you try to lift it out of the water) you will begin to see just what you are up against.

Getting back alongside

There are various methods suggested for getting back alongside the casualty. Each has its virtues, and the better at steering and sailing you are, the greater choice you will have should the time ever come. The simplest is that recommended by Britain's Royal Yachting Association, as part of the Competent Crew courses (which I strongly recommend any new cruising crew to take).

As soon as the alarm is raised, throw one of the lifebelts mounted on the pushpit to the person in the water: if he can swim to it the lifebelt will keep him afloat (and, even more important, provide heartwarming reassurance – take it from one who has been there). If he has a problem – such as being unconscious – it will help mark where he is in the water.

Next, one person must take charge, and the others must keep quiet, pay attention and do what they are told. The one person will be the skipper unless the skipper is the one who has gone overboard: if that is so then the next most experienced crew member should take charge.

One person must be ordered to watch and point at the person in the water: ideally, that is all that person should do, leaving the others to sail the boat. That way, there is least chance of losing sight of the casualty.

As quickly as possible, turn the boat so that she is sailing with the burgee blowing at right

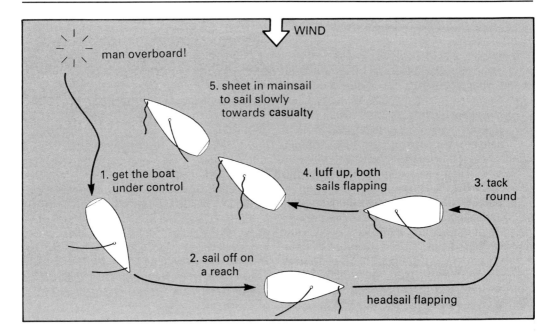

angles across the boat – sailing on a reach, in other words. Sail like that a little distance, letting the headsail flap, and using only the mainsail.

Tack the boat, bringing the headsail across, but letting it flap again. Let the mainsail right out, and point the boat straight at the person in the water. If the mainsail fills, steer away in the direction the burgee is pointing and sail downwind for two or three boat lengths; then try again.

As soon as you can point the boat at the casualty with both sails flapping, sheet-in the mainsail and begin to sail very slowly towards the casualty. It is very important to get the boat slowed down or even stopped at this stage: you can always sheet-in and speed up again, but there is no point arriving back at the person in the water with too much speed on and no way to stop.

You will now find yourself able to make the approach sailing at about 50 or 60 degrees to the wind, nice and slowly and in complete control. Aim to stop about six feet dead to windward of the person in the water. The boat will drift slowly down alongside them.

Using the engine

Another method that is often suggested is the so-called 'quick-stop'. As soon as the person falls in, or the alarm is raised, whoever is steering just shoves the helm down (pushes the tiller away) and tacks the boat, all-standing – in other words without anyone touching any of the sheets. This will have the effect of leaving the boat sailing on the other tack with the headsail hauled back, on the wrong side. This is called 'hove-to' and is a tried and accepted method of keeping any sailing vessel stopped in the water but under more control than if the sails are simply allowed to flog.

From this position you can then work out what to do next, with the advantage that you will be a lot nearer whoever has fallen in.

You might now start the engine – but *make sure it is not in gear*. Having the engine running, even if you do the entire recovery under sail, gives another string to your bow, another option to use should you need it.

If you decide to use the engine to motor to the person in the water, *check and double-check there are no ropes dangling over the side*. It is in the heat of just this sort of moment that normal routines go by the board. The sails are dropped hurriedly, nothing tidied-up, the engine started, the gear level shoved into Ahead – and a moment later the engine stops, a rope wound around the propeller shaft. Now you are in real trouble, with one person in the water and the yacht immobilised: you cannot use the engine and you cannot re-hoist the sails, since it is probably the mainsheet itself which is round the propeller.

If you do use the engine, remember the dangers of coming alongside a person in the water with those terrible propeller blades chopping away just inches from the casualty's legs and feet. Approach very slowly, and as soon as you are within reach of the victim, knock the engine out of gear. As soon as the casualty is secured with a line, stop the engine.

Getting him on board
Rule One: get a line attached to the person in the water right away. That way he is in permanent contact with the boat again. If he can help himself, this will be relatively easy; if he is semi-conscious, it will obviously be difficult. Do not be tempted to use a lassoo-type arrangement with a sliding knot which can tighten round the casualty's chest, or even throat. By now, those on deck should have got into their own safety harnesses, so they do not go in accidentally while working overside with the person in the water.

Should another person go in on purpose, to assist the casualty? It depends on the circumstances. *On no account should the person in command do so*, even if he is the most competent and strongest person and the best swimmer. Once in the water he will become no more than another casualty. If anyone is going to go in to help the casualty, it must not be the person whose greatest contribution can be made by staying on deck, and in charge.

In theory, there are several ways of getting someone back on board. Here are some of them.
• *Using the rubber dinghy*. Good if the dinghy is stowed on deck, already inflated. Slow if the dinghy has to be blown up first, but even so do not reject the idea out of hand. In reality, a rubber dinghy can be inflated in about three minutes. As long as the casualty can be kept afloat and alongside in the meantime this might still be the quickest way. Secure the dinghy painter well forward on the yacht, so the dinghy lies alongside. Get into the dinghy and heave or help the person in the water into the dinghy, then up over the yacht toerail and under the guardrails. If the guardrails have a gate for boarding, this is the obvious place to work.

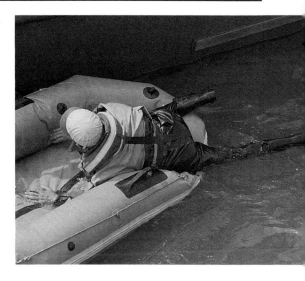

⌂ *If the dinghy is only partly inflated it is easier to scramble into.*

• *Using a boarding ladder*. Fine if the person can climb. The usual place for a boarding ladder on modern boats is on the stern, which is just about the worst place if the yacht is pitching in any sort of sea. The best place, if the boarding ladder can be shifted, is amidships: here any waves passing under the yacht will come nearest the toerail, and can be used to help lift the casualty on board.
• *Using the end of the mainsheet*. The block-and-tackle of the mainsheet can be unshackled at its lower end and, using the boom held up by the topping lift and swung out over the side, used as a lifting tackle. Probably easier and simpler is:
• *Using the main halyard*. Lower the mainsail and stow it roughtly out of the way, on the other side of the yacht to the casualty. Unshackle the main halyard and attach it to the line you have round the casualty. Put the halyard on the halyard winch, or if possible on the main genoa sheet winch, which will be more powerful, and winch him on board. Obviously, the more people you have assisting the casualty, the less chance of injuring him.

All in all, losing someone overboard is a very alarming prospect, and deserves careful thought before it happens. The more familiar you become with the yacht's gear and equipment, the more use you will be should such an emergency occur.

FIRE

Fire on board a small boat can be both terrifying and terminal: it can spread so quickly, leaving no place of safety, that prevention is paramount. We saw in Chapter One that as soon as you come on board you should find out, or be shown, where all the emergency equipment is stowed, and how it is to be used. This includes the fire extinguishers and fire blanket.

The three ingredients of fire

Fire has three ingredients: without any one of them it cannot start, and once started if it can be deprived of even one of the ingredients it will go out. Those three ingredients are fuel, heat and oxygen (which for our purposes simply means air). The swiftest and surest way to deal with a fire is to concentrate on removing first one of the ingredients, then the other two.

Smothering

The most likely place for a fire is probably in the galley, on the top of the stove, and the front-line and often most effective means of dealing with it is the fire blanket. You should find this stowed on a bulkhead near at hand, with instructions for use clearly displayed. Smothering any fire deprives it of oxygen and quickly puts it out, so the same technique can be used for a small fire in, for example, bedding. Smothering is the quickest and surest way of dealing with any small and localised fire – provided you can smother the whole fire.

Extinguishers

Two types of extinguisher are commonly found (should be found) on board: water and dry powder. Contrary to popular belief water is not a universal antidote to fire: in some cases it is almost as dangerous to douse a fire with water as it would be to spray it with paraffin or petrol.

Fires which involve liquid (such as burning fat, paraffin from a heater, or burning diesel fuel on an engine exhaust) should never be hit with water, especially water under pressure (as from an extinguisher). At the least the water will spread the blazing fuel further round the boat, dramatically so if it is squirted rather than merely poured; at the worst, if the fire is really going, the water will be instantaneously converted to steam, possibly causing an explosion.

The dry powder extinguisher works like the fire blanket, by smothering the fire and depriving it of oxygen. It is more effective than the blanket over a wider area, or when a fire has started in an awkward place which a blanket will not completely cover. If in doubt about what is burning, use a powder extinguisher.

The water extinguisher deprives the fire of a different ingredient: heat. It puts out whatever is burning by dramatically cooling it. Use it on solids (bedding, furniture etc) where the fire has got such a good hold by the time you get there that it is too big or well-established to be put out just by smothering.

Aim the extinguisher at the base of the fire – the point where the flames are coming from – and squeeze or press the trigger. A short burst may be enough, since fire extinguishers are remarkably effective, but do not simply put the extinguisher back where you found it. A half-discharged extinguisher tends to lose pressure and become useless, so it must be replaced.

Automatic systems

Some yachts have an automatic system, often in the engine compartment. This uses a third type of extinguisher which discharges an inert gas that smothers the fire. If necessary you can fire the automatic system by hand, usually by hitting a prominent red knob. Obviously such a system can only work in an enclosed, sealed space, so if you ever have to use it remember to give the gas time to smother the fire before opening the engine compartment to see if the fire is out.

⇨ *An engine fire extinguisher.*

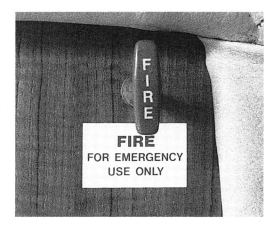

Glossary

Bear away Steering away from the wind.

Beating Zig-zagging (tacking) upwind.

Bolt-rope The rope sewn into the front edge (luff) of a sail.

Burgee The small flag that indicates the wind direction.

Clew The bottom aft corner of a sail.

Guardrails The 'fence' around the deck, supported by stanchions.

Guy A line that stabilises a spinnaker or headsail pole.

Gybe Turning the boat away from the wind so that the wind blows from the other side, causing the sails to flip across.

Halyard A line used to raise a sail.

Head The top corner of a sail; the nautical name for the toilet.

Headsail Any sail that is set in front of the mast on the forestay, such as a genoa, jib or storm jib.

Jackstay The wire or strap running along the side deck which takes the clip of your safety harness line.

Jib A small to medium-sized headsail.

Leech The aft edge of a sail.

Luff The fore edge of a sail; the action of steering the boat up into the wind.

Mainsail The sail set behind the mast, on the boom.

Pulpit The safety frame in the bow of the boat (a similar frame in the stern is known as a pushpit).

Reaching Sailing across the wind. Luffing into the wind puts the boat on a close reach, while bearing away puts her on a broad reach.

Reefing Reducing the area of a sail.

Running Sailing directly downwind, i.e. with the wind blowing from aft.

Running backstays Paired backstays that can be slackened off so they do not foul the boom.

Sheet A line that controls the angle of the sail to the wind.

Shrouds The wires at the sides of the boat that support the mast.

Stays The wires from the bow and stern that support the mast.

Stopper A lever-action device used to jam a line.

Tack The bottom front corner of a sail.

Toerail The shallow ridge that runs around the edge of the deck.

Topping lift A line used to support the boom or spinnaker pole from the masthead.

Warp A mooring line.

Cut off the fuel

Immediately a fire starts, cut off its fuel supply. If it is a heater gone ablaze, for instance, turn off the gas or paraffin; likewise a fire in the galley, or one involving fuel oil. If it is in a cabin, among clothes or bedding, quickly pull away all the combustible material, such as sleeping bags and clothes bags. In a galley fire, turning off the gas instantly deprives the fire both of more fuel and any more of that other ingredient, heat.

Remember the three ingredients of the fire: fuel, heat and air – and work swiftly to remove first one, then the other two.

DISTRESS FLARES AND LIFERAFTS

The skipper should acquaint you, as soon as you are on board, with where the flares are kept and how to operate them; likewise the liferaft. You should make sure you know how to work them.

For reasons best known to the pyrotechnics industry there is no standard method of operating a flare: different makes use different methods so it is important to become familiar with the ones aboard the boat you are on. The moment when you need them, in the dark, when you are cold, wet, frightened and in grave danger, is no time to start trying to read instruction labels.

Types of flare

A rocket flare shoots bright lights up into the sky; you use them when well offshore to alert anyone who may be just over the horizon. Hand flares are for inshore waters and for use at close quarters. They give out either a dense cloud of smoke (for use in daylight) or a bright burning light (for use at night).

Rocket flares are usually fired by pulling a ring on the bottom of the flare; hand flares are usually ignited by striking a flint (which is kept inside a cap at the lower end) over the striker pad on the top of the flare (which is usually protected by a plastic cap which, naturally enough, you have first to remove). Both types of flare are kept in tough, heat-sealed plastic bags (to keep them safe and dry) which, like plastic packaging the world over, yields up its treasure only with reluctance.

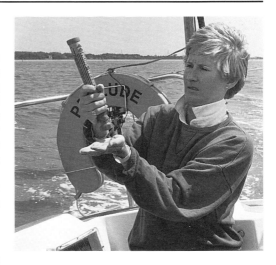

◇ Find out how to fire the flares properly.

Flares are dangerous. Point them away from other people, hold them high and if possible outside the boat, and turn your own face away as you fire them.

Liferafts

The yacht may carry an automatically inflating liferaft for the ultimate emergency. Although the decision to take to it will hardly be yours, it should be made only when there really is no alternative. A yacht even half afloat is a safer, more comfortable place than a flexible rubber raft being flung around by the sea and blown, totally out of control, by the wind. All the same, you should know how to deploy the raft if you have to.

◇ A canister-type liferaft stowed on deck.

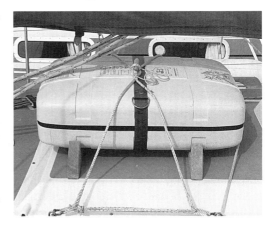